1999–2000
Medical Student's Guide to Successful Residency Matching

1999–2000

Medical Student's Guide to Successful Residency Matching

Lee T. Miller, MD

Director, Pediatric Residency Training Program
Ahmanson Pediatric Center
Cedars-Sinai Medical Center
Professor of Pediatrics
UCLA School of Medicine
Los Angeles, California

Leigh G. Donowitz, MD

Chair, Pediatric Residency Selection Committee
The Children's Medical Center
Professor of Pediatrics
University of Virginia School of Medicine
Charlottesville, Virginia

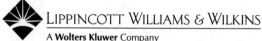

LIPPINCOTT WILLIAMS & WILKINS
A **Wolters Kluwer** Company

Philadelphia · Baltimore · New York · London
Buenos Aires · Hong Kong · Sydney · Tokyo

Acquisitions Editor: Elizabeth A. Nieginski
Editorial Director of Development: Julie P. Scardiglia
Senior *Managing Editor:* Amy G. Dinkel
Marketing Manager: Jennifer Conrad
Compositor: Peirce Graphic Services, Inc.
Printer: Vicks Lithograph & Printing Corp.

9 8 7 6 5 4 3 2 1

Library of Congress Cataloging-in-Publication Data.

Contents

Preface

There are over 25,000 individuals attempting to gain residency training in the United States, and such individuals are faced with the enormous task of selecting from a wide variety of graduate medical education training programs. It is our goal to guide the applicant through the year-long matching process with a step-by-step guide to successful residency matching from start to finish. The scope of this book encompasses specialty selection, curriculum planning for the third and fourth years of medical school, program selection for residency application, strategies for interviewing and ranking, tips for the foreign medical graduate, and an overview of the different matching programs, with particular emphasis on the National Resident Matching Program (NRMP).

We wish to acknowledge the many medical students and house officers whose questions and suggestions have guided us through the writing of this text. In particular, we would like to thank the thousands of students across the country from the Class of 1991 through the Class of 1999, whose enthusiastic comments, suggestions, and questions have helped us strengthen this project. This book was written with the spirit and hope that we can help tomorrow's house officers match successfully with the residency programs of their choosing.

Lee T. Miller, MD
Leigh G. Donowitz, MD

Acknowledgments

We express our sincere appreciation to the following individuals who contributed greatly to the preparation of this text: Alice Cherian, Anne Crowley, PhD, Lynn Elliott, Sylvia Etzel, Charlotte Myers, Kate Perkins, MD, PhD, Ann Thomas Rall, Louisa Shaw, Phyllis Weiland, Tim Wright, MD, and Sharon Young, MD.

In addition, we express our particular gratitude to Liz Lostumbo of the National Resident Matching Program, and to August Colenbrander, MD and Douglas Perry for their tremendous contributions and support.

Choosing Your
Medical Specialty

INTRODUCTION

The aim of this chapter is to provide some guidance to you, the student who remains undecided about which specialty to choose. Of more than 300 medical students who participated in a nationwide survey on specialty choice, 81% considered their choice of specialty to be the most important decision they made during medical school. Of these same students, 80% believed that they did not have enough information on which to base this decision and, as a result, 50% of students postponed this important decision until their fourth year of medical school (1). We suggest additional comprehensive references on this subject in the Recommended Reading list provided in Chapter 10.

Choosing which medical specialty to pursue is a career decision that may carry with it a lifetime commitment to care for specific patients with specific diseases. Some specialists will only deliver babies, only see children, only psychoanalyze, only read radiographs, only examine skin, or only examine eyes. These different specialties also carry with them a certain professional identity that may influence such things as lifestyle and friends, particularly in this time of rapid change in our health care world. Be certain that you take the time to find advisors at all levels in their careers who can describe the profession today and, it is hoped, project for you where that profession may be tomorrow.

ADVISORS FOR SPECIALTY DECISION-MAKING

As a medical student, you may have family members who can provide you with historical and current information on different medical specialties. This advice may be extremely useful because these individuals may well be able to incorporate your background and personality into the discussion. However, this advice can also be extremely pressured and biased. When a parent or family member has strong feelings about your choice of specialty, the counsel may be a detriment to your freedom of decision-making. It is important that you make your own decision, realizing that parental and family disappointments now will disappear in the future with a happier son or daughter who has fulfilled his or her own goals.

Alumni of your school or its residency programs who teach or practice in the area may be extremely useful advisors. They may better understand your educational background and can speak freely of their own decisions and whether their goals have been realized.

Present house officers and chief residents in particular specialties are usually wonderful advisors because they can very accurately reflect on their recent decision-making. They can also comment on the pros and cons of the specific and current residency training requirements and potential employment opportunities upon completion of training.

The Dean of Students may be a good advisor on specialty choice, but is unlikely to be able to offer much specific information on residency programs in a particular discipline unless he or she is specifically trained in that field.

A faculty advisor can be extremely helpful, but again, becomes more useful when you are asking about this advisor's own field of expertise. It is more important to utilize the experience of the faculty advisor after you have chosen a specialty and are seeking more information on that career, residency training, and specific training programs within that particular specialty (see Chapter 4).

REALITIES OF YOUR SPECIALTY CHOICE

It is extremely important that you fully understand the training requirements, the career possibilities, and the lifestyle realities of the specialty you are considering.

Requirements. The minimum training requirements to meet Board eligibility in most specialties are outlined in Table 1.1. Individual program requirements may differ from these minimum Board requirements, including additional years of clinical work and/or research. Programs in family practice, pediatrics, and internal medicine appear to have a shorter training period (usually 3 years) when compared with the surgical subspecialties. However, if you decide to subspecialize (e.g., in pediatric cardiology), training will be 6 years (3 years of pediatric training plus 3 years of pediatric cardiology fellowship). This training period, then, is not very different from the length of time required to complete general surgery training. The Directory of Graduate Medical Education Programs lists requirements for specialty and subspecialty training in all fields (2).

TABLE 1.1
Training Requirements by Specialty*

Specialty	Required Preliminary Track Training (years)	Minimum Required Length of Specialty Residency Training for Board Eligibility (years)	Minimum Total Number of Years of Training to Meet Board Eligibility Requirements	Application Deadline
Anesthesiology	1 (Optional for some Anesthesiology programs)	3	4	Apply to Anesthesiology programs in the fall 2 years before beginning your training in Anesthesiology
Colon and Rectal Surgery	5 (General Surgery)	1	6	Apply to Colon and Rectal Surgery programs 1–2 years before beginning your training in Colon and Rectal Surgery
Dermatology	1	3	4	Apply to Dermatology programs 2 years before beginning your training in Dermatology
Emergency Medicine	1 (Optional for some Emergency Medicine programs)	3	3	Apply to EM programs in the fall 2 years in advance if applying for preliminary training first; otherwise, apply 1 year in advance if EM program incorporates an internship

Family Practice	0	3	3	Apply to Family Practice programs in the fall 1 year before beginning your training in Family Practice
Internal Medicine	0	3	3	Apply to Internal Medicine programs in the fall 1 year before beginning your training in Internal Medicine
Neurology[1] (Adult)	1 (> 8 months Internal Med)	3	4	An early match; apply to Neurology programs 2 years before beginning your training in Adult Neurology
Neurology[2] (Child)	1–2 (Pediatrics and/or Research year)	3	5	Apply to Child Neurology programs 2 years before beginning your training in Child Neurology
Neurosurgery	1	5	6	An early match; apply to Neurosurgery programs 2 years before beginning your training in the neurosurgical sciences

[1]Adult Neurology has a "Two-Tier Match" designed to serve those students who are ready to choose Neurology in January of their senior year as well as those who wish to postpone their decision until January of their PGY-1 year.
[2]Pediatric Neurology positions are filled by direct appointments and not through a matching process.

TABLE 1.1—*continued*

Specialty	Required Preliminary Track Training (years)	Minimum Required Length of Specialty Residency Training for Board Eligibility (years)	Minimum Total Number of Years of Training to Meet Board Eligibility Requirements	Application Deadline
Nuclear Medicine	2	2	4	Apply for Nuclear Medicine during your preliminary track clinical training 1–2 years in advance; apply directly to the program; not a match
Obstetrics-Gynecology	1 (Optional)	3 or 4	4	Apply to OB-GYN programs in the fall 1 year in advance if applying to a 4-year OB-GYN program
Ophthalmology	1	3	4	An early match; apply to Ophthalmology programs 2 years before beginning your training in Ophthalmology
Orthopedic Surgery	1 (Optional for some Orthopedic Surgery programs)	4	5	Apply to Orthopedic Surgery programs in the fall, usually 2 years before beginning your training in Orthopedic Surgery

Specialty				
Otolaryngology	1–2	4	5	An early match; apply to Otolaryngology programs in the fall 2 years before beginning your training in Otolaryngology (or 3 years for programs requiring 2 years of General Surgery training)
Pathology (Combined Anatomical and Clinical)	0	5	5	Apply to Pathology programs in the fall 1 year before beginning your training in Pathology
Pediatrics	0	3	3	Apply to Pediatrics programs in the fall 1 year before beginning your training in Pediatrics
Physical Medicine and Rehabilitation	1 (Optional for some Physical Medicine and Rehabilitation programs)	3–4	4	Apply to PM and R programs in the fall 1 year in advance if going into program which incorporates preliminary training
Plastic Surgery[3]	3 (General Surgery)	2	5	Apply to Plastic Surgery programs in the fall 2 years before beginning your Plastic Surgery training

[3]Some plastic surgery positions are offered at the PGY-1 level through the NRMP Match. These positions are "integrated" and provide 3 years of General Surgery training and 2 years of Plastic Surgery training. Most positions in Plastic Surgery are filled in a separate match in May of the PGY-2 year or later (14 months before the start of Plastic Surgery training).

TABLE 1.1—*continued*

Specialty	Required Preliminary Track Training (years)	Minimum Required Length of Specialty Training Residency Training for Board Eligibility (years)	Minimum Total Number of Years of Training to Meet Board Eligibility Requirements	Application Deadline
Preventive Medicine	1	1	2 (Residency must be followed by a year of field work to meet Board eligibility requirements)	Apply directly to Preventive Medicine programs in the fall 1 year before beginning your preliminary year training
Psychiatry	1	3	4	Apply to Psychiatry programs in the fall 1 year in advance if program includes preliminary training; otherwise, in the fall, 2 years before beginning your training in Psychiatry
Radiology	1 (Optional for some Radiology programs)	4	5	Apply to Radiology programs in the fall 2 years before beginning your training in Radiology

Specialty				Application timing
Surgery	0	5	5	Apply to General Surgery programs in the fall 1 year before beginning your training in Surgery
Thoracic Surgery	5 (General Surgery Residency)	2	7	Apply to Thoracic Surgery programs in the fall 2 years before beginning your training in Thoracic Surgery
Urology	1–2	3–4	5	An early match; apply to Urology programs in the fall 2–3 years before beginning your training in Urology

Note: Individual program requirements may differ from these minimum board requirements, including additional years of clinical work and/or research.

Career Opportunities. Consideration of the availability of positions upon completion of training is a necessary part of this decision. It is important to determine whether opportunities will be available to practice your academic or private specialty, or whether a given field is already too competitive and saturated.

Lifestyle. An accurate assessment of what effect your career choice will have on your personal lifestyle is also imperative. Weekly hours, nighttime and weekend duties, geographic location, financial compensation, and many other lifestyle factors will be greatly influenced by this career decision. It is important to envision as much of this as possible and truthfully acknowledge your own personal needs and priorities as you make this decision (1).

Once you have sorted through the above, keep in mind that the future of many specialties is impossible to predict. Many of the medical fields have markedly changed in the last 20–30 years and may continue to do so. Radiology, for example, is a field that has enjoyed tremendous growth. The radiologist is no longer limited to just the black and white roentgenogram. This discipline now includes subspecialties in angiography, ultrasonography, nuclear magnetic resonance imaging, and nuclear scanning. The primary care specialties have undergone the most impressive growth. Although future changes in specialties are difficult to predict, one's own personal preferences will probably not change radically with time. Therefore, the rotations in which you are most comfortable during your third and fourth years probably reflect an environment that you will enjoy for a long time. This "gut feeling" of comfort should carry significant weight in your decision-making.

SPECIALTY COMPETITION

It is important to determine your competitiveness or "how good you look" compared with the rest of your class and other students competing for similar positions from all over the country. If you are a superb student at a small, relatively little known school, and if you can obtain excellent letters of reference, and if you have strong interview skills showing your directedness and dedication, then you should apply to your top choices regardless of how competitive these medical centers or specialties may be. If you are in the middle of your class even at a renowned institution, you will need strong letters of recommendation and excellent interviews to obtain your top choices. It is important, however, that you list your strengths and weaknesses and understand your class rank and competitiveness so that you neither underestimate nor overestimate your abilities.

It is also important that you assess the competitiveness of the programs to which you are applying. Some specialties have many unfilled places each year, and, in these fields, you should not be afraid to aim high for a strong residency position. We recommend that you apply to excellent programs where your chances of securing a position are not high but still possible, and have other places on your list that are good, solid, but less competitive programs where you have a higher likelihood of successful matching. The matching system, as it is established, allows you to do better, if possible, than you would through a routine acceptance situation, particularly in the less competitive specialties. In highly competitive programs, it is much more important to assess your class standing very accurately and have the chairman or a faculty member with expertise in this specialty honestly assess your likelihood of success in securing a residency position in this field. Particularly in specialties with very small numbers of positions (e.g., dermatology, orthopedics, and neurosurgery), it is extremely important to find out if you are competitive for one of these positions.

It is suggested that you be well along in this career decision-making process by the early fall of your senior year.

OTHER TIPS FOR SPECIALTY SELECTION

For those of you who find yourselves during the summer of 1999 still not knowing which career direction you'd like to pursue, we'd like to urge you to relax! It may become increasingly more difficult for you to maintain your composure while more and more friends share with you their excitement over their own career decisions. Please remember that this is not a race and your time will come soon enough. There are, however, several things we can suggest that might help you to get there sooner rather than later.

Most importantly, we urge you to take advantage of the flexibility of your senior year to reexplore specialty areas that you may be considering. This is your chance to "retest the waters" before making your final decisions. You may have a very different impression when you "revisit" a service as a senior student on an elective or subinternship. You will likely no longer share the worries of the third-year students on your service (e.g., presentations on rounds, preparations for final exams) and can focus your energies instead on trying to feel what it would be like to dedicate your career to that particular specialty.

If you're considering more than one specialty during the summer of 1999, you might also want to write for information from more than one type of residency training program. Often, when learning in greater detail about the specifics of each training program, students may find themselves pulled in one direction rather than another, and also find themselves more excited about a particular type of training program. Once you do make your specialty choice, you'll be ready to complete the application materials in a timely fashion, having already solicited materials from programs earlier in your decision-making process.

While some students look for as many reasons as possible to put off writing their personal statement, we might even suggest that you consider more than one—that is, a different personal statement for each specialty area you're considering. Many students have found this to be an extremely revealing exercise when they have difficulty articulating on paper all of the reasons why they might want to pursue specialty "A" versus the ease with which they can explain on paper all of the reasons for pursuing specialty "B".

Regardless of how and when you choose which specialty you'd like to pursue, we can't emphasize enough how important it is that you and you alone make this decision. You're the one who will have to roll out of bed at 5:30 or 6:00 in the morning to prepare for work rounds, not your many friends or family members who are urging you to pursue various directions. Once again, the bottom line here is that only you can make this decision from your heart!

REFERENCES

1. Stein J. Impact on personal life key to choosing a medical specialty in the '80's. *Internal Medicine World Report* 1988; 3:7.
2. American Medical Association. *Directory of Graduate Medical Education Programs.* Chicago, American Medical Association, annual publication.

Planning Your Clinical Years

THE JUNIOR YEAR—CLERKSHIP SCHEDULING

Many sophomore medical students will be given the opportunity to bid on the sequence of their junior clinical clerkships. We'd like to stress that the order of your rotations will ultimately have little impact upon your overall performance, and that there are advantages and disadvantages to starting on more or less rigorous services. However, if you're approaching your junior year with a particular "favorite specialty" in mind, it may be in your best interest to avoid doing this specialty rotation at the very start of your third year. Remember that your first weeks to months on the wards will be spent "learning the ropes" of the clinical clerk, including presentations, histories and physicals, venipuncture and other procedures, and learning your way around the hospital. Although by no means a hard-and-fast rule, you are much more likely to "shine" a bit later in your junior year when you are more polished and comfortable with your new clinical responsibilities. Similarly, some students advocate avoiding their favorite clerkships at the very end of the junior year when they are more likely to be burned out and exhausted from the rigors of the preceding 9–12 months. However, we'd like to emphasize again that regardless of the sequence of your clinical clerkships, you will have multiple opportunities to demonstrate your abilities and to perform them admirably.

THE JUNIOR YEAR—CLERKSHIP LOCATIONS

Most medical schools will offer their students opportunities to rotate through services at either a home institution (usually a university hospital) or multiple affiliated centers, which may vary from tertiary care centers, to community hospitals, to outlying clinics, to Veterans' Administration hospitals, to county facilities. Regardless of your clerkship assignments, the most important thing is to strive for excellence on your clinical rotations. You will undoubtedly face several non-ideal and otherwise difficult situations along the way. For example, a poor attending, a weak resident, or a county health care facility with poorly funded ancillary services may present obstacles. Despite this, you will do yourself a disservice by allowing your environment to affect your attitude adversely and, thus, to result in less than your best performance. Furthermore, if you feel slighted that you have missed an opportunity to work with the faculty at your home institution in your specialty of interest, you will have ample occasions to demonstrate your abilities on elective opportunities throughout your senior year.

THE SENIOR YEAR—REQUIRED ROTATIONS, ELECTIVE TIME, EXTRAMURAL ELECTIVES, AND INTERVIEW SCHEDULING

Be sure to check with your dean's office for a list of required rotations for your senior year. At the same time, you may inquire as to the maximum number of rotations that may be taken away from your home institution. In most instances, the majority of your last year of medical school may be spent on clinical, research, or reading electives. Your senior year should not be perceived as unimportant just because it affords flexibility and the opportunity to pursue elective training. This year should be viewed as a valuable opportunity to solidify your clinical skills and fund of knowledge and to broaden your foundation in medicine. Be sure to discuss your plans and elective choices well in advance with your faculty advisor, and perhaps with other more senior students who are preparing for graduation. In planning your senior schedule, you should allocate 2–4 weeks of "free time" for interviewing. This interview period should preferably be after November 1 when your dean's letter of recommendation has already been mailed out. Most elective supervisors and attending physicians will understand if you request additional days off for interviewing at other times during the late fall or winter. We also recommend a light schedule filled with less rigorous electives at the end of your senior year (i.e., after Match Day). You will enjoy having more leisure time to relax and unwind before your internship and will appreciate a lighter schedule as you begin making plans for finding a new home, packing, and moving.

An "acting internship" or "subinternship" in your specialty of choice will significantly add to your credentials and strengthen your recommendation if you perform admirably. Such rotations are not only excellent teaching opportunities, but also "confidence builders" as you approach the end of medical school and the beginning of your internship. At the same time, it is crucial to maintain a sense of balance throughout your senior year by rotating through multiple disciplines. Do not try to mimic your internship as a senior student by taking more than two or possibly three electives in your specialty of choice. Rather, we recommend that you take advantage of this valuable elective time in multiple disciplines to broaden your foundation in clinical medicine. For example, a critical care rotation will help all students improve their organizational skills and expertise with procedures. Similarly, a rotation on a radiology service, in an emergency room, or on an anesthesiology service should provide valuable teaching for all students pursuing any kind of clinical training. "Extramural electives" or "audition electives" (i.e., electives at institutions other than your medical school or its closely affiliated centers) can either help or hinder your application for residency at that center. A less than strong performance at another institution will markedly lessen your chances for matching at that institution. We do not recommend extramural rotations solely for the purpose of impressing a residency selection committee unless your faculty advisor believes that it is in your best interest for a particularly competitive specialty or program. If you are a superb student, you will likely be able to match in one of the programs of your choosing without rotating there on an extramural elective. On the other hand, rotations at other institutions provide tremendous opportunities to:

- Learn more about a particular type of institution (e.g., rotating through a children's hospital versus a general university hospital versus a community hospital).
- Learn more about a particular geographic area in which you're considering relocating for your internship.
- Learn more about a particular discipline on a stronger teaching service than your home institution can offer (e.g., rotat-

ing on a strong hematology-oncology service with a fine reputation for teaching at a medical school across town) (1).

We also recommend that you take advantage of the many unique opportunities afforded to senior medical students (e.g., rotations in Alaska, developing nations, or Great Britain) provided your overall curriculum is well balanced and meets all requirements for graduation. Many medical schools will assign a faculty advisor to counsel students on international elective opportunities and exchange programs, as well as direct students toward resources for funding.

In summary, your senior year offers tremendous opportunities to broaden your knowledge base in multiple disciplines while allowing you to sort out and solidify career choices and to explore internship opportunities. Elective planning should be carefully reviewed and discussed with your faculty advisor as you embark on this exciting and enriching last year of your undergraduate medical education.

CLASS OF 2000 TIMETABLE

It's critical that you understand the application timetable as you plan your senior schedules. For example, for most specialties you will need to have a dedicated block of time between November and January for interviews, and most students block out 2–4 weeks of vacation between November and January for this purpose. However, for a small subset of specialties, the entire application, interview, and ranking processes occur early (i.e., *Early Match Specialties*), and you need to plan accordingly so that you get all of your interviews scheduled appropriately. To help you plan effectively for the residency matching process, we have created the following timetable to guide you through your junior and senior years.

APRIL 1999–MAY 1999

- Begin to inquire about "away" electives at other medical schools (optional).
- The American Medical Association's updated computer directory of programs entitled the Fellowship and Residency Electronic Interactive Database Access System (alias AMA–FREIDA) (2) should be available for review through your medical school's Dean of Student Affairs Office.
- Begin meeting with faculty advisors and senior students to discuss planning for your fourth year and the upcoming application process.

JUNE 1999–JULY 1999

- Begin writing away for residency applications.
- Begin requesting letters of recommendation from faculty members (you may also do this earlier in your junior year while memories are fresh from clerkship attendings).
- A student agreement (contract) with National Resident Matching Program must be signed and submitted by all students.
- Applicants to early match specialties (e.g., ophthalmology, neurology, neurosurgery, urology, and otolaryngology) should sign and submit individual agreements to participate in these Match programs.
- Continue to seek individual counseling from faculty, house staff, and internship advisors.
- Application photos should be taken.

AUGUST 1999–SEPTEMBER 1999

- Continue to request application materials.
- Continue individual counseling.
- Continue to be aware of early application deadlines.
- Continue to solicit letters of recommendation from the faculty.
- Be aware that some programs may want supportive documents (i.e., transcripts, Board scores, and letters of recommendation) prior to the November 1 release of your Dean's letter.

- If you feel comfortable that you have decided upon an area of specialization, begin preparing your personal statement. (Do not be anxious if you are still uncertain!)
- If you are applying to one of the PGY-2 (Independent) Matches that offer a Central Application Service (Ophthalmology, Otolaryngology, and Neurosurgery), you should aim to submit your application and supportive documents by mid-September through mid-October.

OCTOBER 1999–NOVEMBER 1999

- Continue to seek advice from faculty, house staff, and internship advisors.
- You should begin mailing out your application materials in October.
- You should now be scheduling interview appointments (the majority of programs will begin interviewing in November, although early match programs may begin as early as September).
- If you are applying for PGY-2 positions (whether they be through the NRMP or through one of the Independent Matching Programs) in addition to PGY-1 positions (through the NRMP), please try to schedule both sets of interviews for the same trip.
- Dean's letters will be released after November 1 as mandated by the Association of American Medical Colleges.
- By mid-November, you might want to follow up on all applications that you have submitted to be sure that your application files are complete.
- Independent applicants should be enrolled with the National Resident Matching Program (NRMP) by late October of 1999.
- "Shared Residency Pair Forms" must be submitted to the NRMP by late October of 1999 for those applicants interested in shared schedule positions.

DECEMBER 1999–JANUARY 2000

- Continue to seek advice from faculty, house staff, and internship advisors.

- Continue the interview process.
- The ranking and matching processes for most early match specialties will likely occur in January of 2000.

FEBRUARY 2000

- Continue to seek advice from faculty, house staff, and internship advisors.
- Complete final interviewing.
- Consider sending follow-up letters to programs (optional).
- Begin preparations to enter your rank list via the World Wide Web, and be sure that you're aware of all deadlines!

MARCH 2000

- The "Scramble Process" for unmatched applicants and unfilled programs begins.
- Independent applicants and U.S. students will be able to access match results via both the NRMP Web Page and the NRMP Voice Response System on Match Day.

REFERENCES

1. Darrow V. The "audition" elective. In Langsley D. (Ed): *How to Select Residents*. Chapter 4. Evanston, IL, American Board of Medical Specialties Publishers, 1988; pp. 49–59.
2. American Medical Association. *Fellowship and Residency Electronic Interactive Database Access System (AMA—FREIDA),* Chicago, American Medical Association, 1998.

The Matching Process

INTRODUCTION

There are generally four different paths of residency application. This chapter outlines the particulars of each one, including the National Resident Matching Program (NRMP), the United States Armed Forces Match, Advanced Specialty Programs with their own matches, and programs that select their residents from a direct application process.

NATIONAL RESIDENT MATCHING PROGRAM (NRMP)

The vast majority of positions for graduate medical training will be filled through the National Resident Matching Program (NRMP). In fact, each year approximately 90% of medical students graduating in the United States use the NRMP to obtain postgraduate training positions. This program offers the applicant the opportunity to rank residency programs independently and confidentially in order of preference. Similarly, residency selection committees are given the opportunity to rank the candidates that have chosen to interview at their institution. The final outcome is that each applicant is matched to the training program highest on the applicant's Rank Order List that has offered the applicant a position. A complete listing of all programs participating in the NRMP is published annually in October in the *NRMP Directory* (1). The purchase price of the *NRMP Directory* for the current year is $35.00 and for prior editions is $25.00. Copies may be ordered by writing directly to:

> National Resident Matching Program
> Attn: Membership and Publication Orders
> 2501 'M' Street
> Washington, DC 20037-1307

Independent applicants may also contact the NRMP by calling (202) 828-0566. There is a separate published number for U.S. seniors, although most communication between U.S. seniors and the NRMP occurs through medical school NRMP coordinators.

Applicants must meet requirements established by the Accreditation Council for Graduate Medical Education to enroll in the National Resident Matching Program. Senior students enrolled in United States medical schools accredited by the Liaison Committee on Medical Education (LCME) who are sponsored by the medical schools are eligible for registration. The same is true for graduates of the schools. All sponsored applicants will receive communications from the NRMP through their Dean of Student Affairs. Independents include students and graduates of Canadian medical schools, students and graduates of schools accredited by the American Osteopathic Association, and graduates of medical schools not so accredited who hold an unrestricted license to practice medicine in a U.S. jurisdiction or who have passed the examinations necessary for certification by the Educational Commission for Foreign Medical Graduates (including "Fifth Pathway" participants). You should consult the *NRMP Handbook for Students* (2) or the *NRMP Handbook of Independent Applicants* (3) for a more detailed description of the rules and regulations of the NRMP. The calendar of important dates for the current match is printed on the back cover of the *NRMP Directory* and should be adhered to. *Deadline dates refer to the date of receipt of materials at the NRMP office.*

Applicants who participate in both the Canadian Resident Matching Service (CaRMS) and the NRMP are expected to accept a position if matched into a Canadian Program. The earlier schedule of CaRMS allows applicants to compete for a Canadian position and, if unsuccessful, continue to participate in the NRMP. The CaRMS informs the NRMP of the dual participants who have matched into a Canadian program, and these individuals are automatically withdrawn from the NRMP match.

CATEGORIES OF MATCHING PROGRAMS WITHIN THE NRMP

The NRMP offers several different categories of matching opportunities, as outlined below. These include categorical programs, preliminary tracks, and advanced specialty programs.

Categorical Programs. Such programs offer positions during the first postgraduate year, with no requirement for previous postgraduate medical education. Most categorical programs are 3–5 years in duration and ultimately lead to eligibility for Board certification upon successful completion of the programs.

Transitional Programs. Formerly known as "flexible internships," transitional year programs provide the resident with 1 year of experience in multiple specialties. For example, this type of residency may include rotations in internal medicine, and/or emergency medicine, general surgery, pediatrics, obstetrics and gynecology, and psychiatry during the first postgraduate year. Transitional year programs are designed to provide broad clinical experience for those physicians who have not yet chosen a given specialty, or for those medical school graduates who think that such experience will provide a strong foundation for subsequent graduate medical education (e.g., anesthesiology and radiology). Information on such programs may be obtained by writing to:

> Executive Director
> Association for Hospital Medical Education
> Council of Transitional Year Program Directors
> 1200 19th Street
> Suite 300
> Washington, DC 20036
> (202) 857-1196

Preliminary Tracks in Internal Medicine, General Surgery, and Pediatrics. Like the transitional year programs, preliminary tracks in internal medicine, general surgery, and, in some cases, pediatrics provide the resident with between 1 and 2 years of PGY-1 (to PGY-2) training in each discipline. Residents applying for such tracks are not seeking Board eligibility in these specialties, but rather 1–2 years of introductory clinical medicine that may serve as a prerequisite for additional postgraduate medical education in other disciplines (e.g., anesthesiology, radiology, and otolaryngology).

Advanced Specialty Programs. These programs begin in the second or third postgraduate year and require 1–2 years of preliminary track training in internal medicine, general surgery, or pediatrics, or 1 year of transitional year training. It should be pointed out that these programs commence the year following the match year, i.e., in 1999 for the 1998 Match. Students ranking such programs are provided the opportunity to link compatible PGY-1 residencies in the same geographical area as the advanced program if a match results. Examples of programs that require such preliminary training include orthopedic surgery, diagnostic and therapeutic radiology, anesthesiology, ophthalmology, dermatology, and some programs in psychiatry and emergency medicine. Some, but not all, institutions will offer candidates 1–2 years of preliminary or transitional track training if accepted into their advanced specialty programs. Applicants to advanced specialty programs may have to complete two Rank Order Lists: one for advanced training programs and a separate supplemental Rank Order List for applications for the PGY 1–2 years.

The above information is summarized in Table 3.1.

SPECIAL MATCHING OPPORTUNITIES WITHIN THE NRMP

The NRMP offers several special matching opportunities to meet the personal or professional needs of some candidates. These include the following:

Shared-Schedule Positions. Some programs will allow two residents to share one full-time position by alternating the months when each house officer is on service. For example, a traditional 3-year primary care training program may take two residents a total of 6 years for both house officers to meet the requirements of Board eligibil-

TABLE 3.1.
Overview of Training Duration in Residencies

1	2	3	4	5	6-7
Family Practice					
Emergency Medicine					
Pediatrics			Subspecialties		+
Internal Medicine			Subspecialties		
Obstetrics/Gynecology					
Pathology			+		
General Surgery				Subspecialties	
	Neurological Surgery				
	Orthopedic surgery				
	Otolaryngology				
	Urology				
Transitional or Prelim Medicine or Prelim Surgery	Anesthesiology				
	Dermatology				
	Neurology				
	Nuclear Medicine				
	Ophthalmology				
	Physical Medicine				
	Psychiatry				
	Radiology–Diagnostic				
	Radiation Oncology				

A sampling of various types of residencies is diagrammed above.
The length of each bar is the period of years of training required for certification by the various Specialty Boards. Many specialties indicated as starting in the PGY-2 year now offer categorical tracks that include the first year. Please refer to the most recent edition of the American Medical Association's *Directory of Graduate Medical Education Programs* (5) for updated official requirements.
Adapted with permission from the NRMP (3).

ity. For the 1998 Match, at the time of publication, of the registered 610 Preliminary (P) programs, of the 2793 Categorical (C) programs, and of the 530 Advanced (S) programs, only 11 programs indicated that they would consider applications for shared-schedule positions. Programs offering such shared schedules are identified in the AMA–FREIDA system (4) and should be contacted directly for specific details. Applicants interested in shared-schedule residency positions must enroll individually in the NRMP. By mid-November, you must also submit a "shared residency pair form" to the NRMP. The guidelines for such registration procedures are clearly outlined in the *NRMP Handbook for Students* (2).

Couples. The NRMP provides the opportunity for any two applicants to rank programs, and ultimately to match with programs in geographic proximity to one another. Each partner applies as an individual, except that the two partners must agree on the geographic parameters that fit their needs. Because of this constraint, individuals who participate in the Match as a couple tend to increase the overall number of programs applied to, in order to maximize the number of interviews secured. Partners must be honest about their choices in two important respects. First, they must consider the competitiveness of each partner with respect to his or her choice of specialty, and be realistic about their chances of matching in their chosen specialty. Second, if a match is impossible in the same location, partners must decide if they would prefer to be matched to different locations, or if one partner would prefer to go unmatched so that the partners can be assured of staying together. Those couples interested in matching together through one of the Independent Matching Programs should contact the Independent Matching Program directly for more information.

Individuals who wish to match as a couple should let programs know of their intention. Depending upon when the decision is made to participate as a couple, partners can inform their programs by a variety of methods, including a cover memo accompanying their application, through their personal statement, and/or during the personal interview. The decision to participate in the Match as a couple must be made by the time rank order lists are submitted in February.

If possible, it is beneficial for partners to interview in the same city at the same time in order to share the experience of the hospitals and the city. Occasionally, only one partner will be invited to interview at a hospital where the specialties of both partners are represented. Because an interview is almost always necessary to rank a program, the invited partner may consider calling the program to request that the partner also be interviewed.

The NRMP has special rank order list forms for couples, which include instructions on how to complete the forms. The rank order list form contains reminders to the participants about the following points: each partner must have the same number of programs; programs must be active in the Match, and an inactive program disqualifies the choice; if one partner withdraws at the last minute, the other's rank order list remains valid and will be used unless he or she notifies the NRMP to the contrary. The special rank order list forms for couples are available in the *NRMP Handbook for Students,* in the *NRMP Handbook for Independent Applicants,* and in the *NRMP Directory.*

At the time that rank order lists are completed, each partner must compile an individual preference list. The partners then "negotiate" compatible lists, and all combinations and permutations must be considered, as outlined in the NRMP's *Instructions for the Completion and Submission of the Couple's Rank Order List of Paired Programs,* as well as the NRMP's *Handbook for Students.* It is during this stage that having interviewed together really helps. Partners should consider setting aside a special time to work on their lists together, perhaps a weekend away from interruptions.

Remember, the "basic rules" apply for couples as well as for the regular match; e.g., a rank order list can only contain

15 distinct programs, otherwise a fee is incurred; do not rank a program if you do not want to go there; and a rank order list can contain various specialties and types (including Categorical, Preliminary, and Supplemental).

In addition to the normal $40.00 NRMP registration fee for U.S. medical students and $90.00 for Independent Applicants, the fee for those applicants matching as a couple is $15.00 per partner, or $30.00 per pair. Also, please be aware that if partners are also applying to Supplemental Programs, supplemental rank order lists cannot be paired.

Combined Training Programs. In recent years there has been a very dramatic increase in the number of combined-specialty resident training opportunities. A complete listing of these programs may be found in the *Directory of Graduate Medical Education Programs* (5) and in the AMA–FREIDA System (4). At this time such training options include the following:

- *Combined Internal Medicine/Emergency Medicine Programs*— These programs offer 5 years of combined training, 2½ years in each specialty, acceptable to both the American Board of Internal Medicine and the American Board of Emergency Medicine toward certification.
- *Combined Internal Medicine/Family Medicine Programs*— The American Board of Internal Medicine and the American Board of Family Practice offer dual certification for candidates who have satisfactorily completed 4 years of combined training in programs approved by both boards.
- *Combined Internal Medicine/Neurology*—These programs offer 5 years of combined training acceptable to both the American Board of Internal Medicine and the American Board of Neurology.
- *Combined Internal Medicine/Pediatrics Programs*—These programs offer 4 years of combined training, 2 years in each specialty, acceptable to both the American Board of Internal

Medicine and the American Board of Pediatrics toward certification.

- *Combined Internal Medicine/Physical Medicine and Rehabilitation*—These programs offer 5 years of combined training, 2½ years in each specialty, acceptable to both the American Board of Internal Medicine and the American Board of Physical Medicine and Rehabilitation toward certification.

- *Combined Internal Medicine/Psychiatry Programs*—These programs offer 5 years of combined training, acceptable to both the American Board of Internal Medicine and the American Board of Psychiatry and Neurology.

- *Combined Neurology/Physical Medicine and Rehabilitation*—These programs offer 5 years of combined training, acceptable to both the American Board of Neurology and the American Board of Physical Medicine and Rehabilitation toward certification. This training must follow a PGY-1 year that meets the requirements for neurology training.

- *Combined Pediatrics/Emergency Medicine Programs*—These programs offer 5 years of combined training, acceptable to both the American Board of Pediatrics and the American Board of Emergency Medicine toward certification.

- *Combined Pediatrics/Physical Medicine and Rehabilitation Programs*—These programs offer 5 years of combined training, acceptable to both the American Board of Pediatrics and the American Board of Physical Medicine and Rehabilitation toward certification.

- *Combined Pediatrics/Psychiatry/Child Psychiatry Programs*—These 5-year programs include 2 years of training in pediatrics, 1½ years of adult psychiatry, and 1½ years of child and adolescent psychiatry.

- *Combined Psychiatry/Family Practice*—The American Board of Family Practice and the American Board of Psychiatry and Neurology offer dual certification in family practice and psychiatry. A combined residency in family practice and psychiatry must include at least 5 years of coherent training integral to residencies in the two disciplines.

- *Combined Psychiatry/Neurology*—The American Board of Psychiatry and Neurology has established guidelines for combined training in Psychiatry and Neurology. A combined residency must include postgraduate year one (PGY-1) training that is acceptable to neurology, plus a minimum of 5 years of combined residency training. The 5 years of residency training are usually taken at one approved institution, but may be taken at no more than two approved institutions.

· *Combined Surgery/Plastic Surgery*—These programs are integrated programs where residents are matched directly into plastic surgery. Their 5 years of combined training may include some plastic surgery rotations during the first 3 years of their general surgery training.

For more information regarding any of the preceding training opportunities, you may contact the Specialty Board offices or may address your questions to the program directors at each individual institution.

THE UNITED STATES ARMED FORCES PROGRAMS

The Army, Navy, and Air Force have their own graduate medical education training programs that do not participate in the National Resident Matching Program. Applicants to such training programs must be qualified for appointment as commissioned officers in the Armed Services. Positions may be filled by graduates of accredited schools of medicine and osteopathic medicine, or by United States graduates of non-United States and non-Canadian medical schools, provided they are certified by the Educational Commission for Foreign Medical Graduates. Most first-year graduate medical education positions in the Armed Services are filled by individuals with existing active duty service obligations. We recommend that applicants to the Armed Services program apply to the NRMP as well, as there are often fewer spaces available than the number of applicants vying for military positions. You must then withdraw your application from the civilian match when you receive a military appointment, which occurs several months in advance of civilian "Match Day." Your withdrawal from the NRMP must occur in advance of the NRMP deadline for the submission of Rank Order Lists. For additional information, contact your local Armed Services recruitment officer.

ADVANCED SPECIALTY PROGRAMS WITH THEIR OWN MATCHING PROGRAMS

There are some specialties that have established their own matching programs for resident selection. Please note that some specialties offer training positions through *both* the NRMP and through the independent matching process, and we recommend consulting with your medical school Dean of Student Affairs office for an updated list of such programs.[1] At present the following specialties have independent matching programs with different timetables for application than the NRMP.

Neurology. For additional information and registration in the neurology matching program, write to:

Neurology Matching Program
P.O. Box 7584
San Francisco, CA 94120-7584
Telephone: (415) 447-0350
FAX: (415) 561-8535
Email: help@sfmatch.org
Web site: www.SFMATCH.org

Note that Neurology has a "two-tier" match. Openings for PGY-2 in 2000 that are not filled in the January 1999 match will be frozen and offered again in the January 2000 match.

Neurosurgery. Applicants to programs in Neurosurgery

---

[1] For the 1998 Match through the NRMP, the number of positions in categorical programs were as follows: 37 in neurological surgery, 32 in neurology, 7 in ophthalmology, 46 in otolaryngology and 49 in plastic surgery.

may use a Central Application Service, completing only one application form and only one set of support documents. For these programs it means that all applications are in a uniform format and that they do not need to spend administrative time assembling applicant files one document at a time. For additional information and registration in the neurosurgery matching program, write to:

Neurological Surgery Matching Program
P.O. Box 7584
San Francisco, CA 94120-7584
Telephone: (415) 447-0350
FAX: (415) 561-8535
Email: help@sfmatch.org
Web site: www.SFMATCH.org

Ophthalmology. Applicants to programs in Ophthalmology must use a Central Application Service. For additional information and registration in the ophthalmology matching program, write to:

Ophthalmology Matching Program
P.O. Box 7584
San Francisco, CA 94120-7584
Telephone: (415) 447-0350
FAX: (415) 561-8535
Email: help@sfmatch.org
Web site: www.SFMATCH.org

Otolaryngology. Applicants to programs in Otolaryngology, like Ophthalmology, must use a Central Application Service. For additional information and registration in the otolaryngology matching program, write to:

Otolaryngology Matching Program
P.O. Box 7584
San Francisco, CA 94120-7584
Telephone:(415) 447-0350

FAX: (415) 561-8535
Email: help@sfmatch.org
Web site: www.SFMATCH.org

Plastic Surgery. While some plastic surgery programs will make "integrated appointments" at the PGY-1 level through the NRMP (offering 3 years of surgery and 2 years of plastic surgery by a single appointment), all other appointments are handled by the Plastic Surgery Matching Program. For more information and registration materials, write to:

Plastic Surgery Matching Program
P.O. Box 7584
San Francisco, CA 94120-7584
Telephone: (415) 447-0350
FAX: (415) 561-8535
Email: help@sfmatch.org
Web site: www.SFMATCH.org

Please note that the Plastic Surgery Matching Program also has its own Central Application Service located in Phoenix, Arizona. You will receive detailed information on this service and its application process when you request information from the Plastic Surgery Matching Program in San Francisco.

Urology. For additional information and registration in the urology matching program, write to:

AUA Residency Matching Program
2425 West Loop South, Suite 333
Houston, TX 77027-4207
e-mail address: resmatch@auanet.org

Each of the above specialty matching programs will provide you with a current timetable for receipt of registration materials and rank lists. Some may provide you with statistics as to the competitiveness of their specialty based upon matching statistics from the previous academic year. Because some of the above specialties are particularly competitive, you might also consider registering with the NRMP with alternative specialty applications in mind. Registration with the NRMP will also be required for application to prerequisite training programs that select their house officers through the NRMP (e.g., 1 or 2 years of general surgery before beginning a training program in neurosurgery or otolaryngology).

NONMATCH PROGRAMS

Although the minority, some graduate training programs do not participate in any matching program, but rather select their residents from a direct application process (e.g., some programs in Oral Surgery). As application procedures may vary from year to year, we suggest that you contact the program directors directly (as outlined in the American Medical Association's *Fellowship and Residency Electronic Interactive Database Access System* or *AMA–FREIDA* system) for specific details on their application process on an annual basis (4).

REFERENCES

1. *NRMP Directory—1999 Match,* National Resident Matching Program, Washington, DC, 1998.
2. *NRMP Handbook for Students,* National Resident Matching Program, Washington, DC, 1998.
3. *NRMP Handbook for Independent Applicants,* National Residency Matching Program, Washington, DC, 1998.
4. American Medical Association. *Fellowship and Residency Electronic Interactive Database Access System (AMA–FREIDA),* Chicago, American Medical Association, 1998.
5. American Medical Association. *Directory of Graduate Medical Education Programs,* American Medical Association, Chicago, annual publication.

Selecting Programs for Application

INTRODUCTION

The first step in selecting programs for application is to review an up-to-date listing of all programs in your specialty of choice that are approved by the Accreditation Council of Graduate Medical Education. A directory of such programs is published annually by the American Medical Association. Prior to March of 1990, hard copies of this directory were distributed through the Dean of Student Affairs offices free of charge to all enrolled senior medical students. Since then, comprehensive information regarding each training program is made available on IBM-compatible diskettes (known as the American Medical Association Fellowship and Residency Electronic Interactive Database Access System, or AMA–FREIDA) (1), which should now be readily accessible to you through the office of the Dean of Student Affairs at your medical school. FREIDA can also be accessed through the American Medical Association's general home page (http: //www.ama-assn.org) under Medical Science and Education. During the summer of 1998, program directors of all accredited specialty and subspecialty programs were asked to enter detailed data on these preprogrammed diskettes, including information on the size of each program, work schedules, call frequency, availability of "shared-schedule positions," required rotations, features of their didactic curriculum, maternity and paternity leave policies, insurance coverage, and vacation policies. This information will be updated on an annual basis. Each program listing will also include the name and address of the current Residency Program Director who will respond to your inquiries. Each summer and fall thousands of medical students send postcards and letters requesting application materials and printed information about each program.

The American Medical Association will continue to publish an annual Directory of Graduate Medical Education Programs (2) (known as the "Green Book") that should be available for your review through the Student Affairs office of your medical school. In addition to providing a complete directory of all accredited residency and fellowship training programs, this hard-copy text will also include the following information that is not currently available in the AMA–FREIDA system: requirements for accreditation of programs; certification requirements in various subspecialties; and an updated statistical report on graduate medical education in the United States. You may order copies of the Directory of Graduate Medical Education by writing directly to:

> Order Department
> American Medical Association
> P.O. Box 109050
> Chicago, IL 60610-9050
> 1-800-621-8335

HOW MANY PROGRAMS?

Most students will request information from a larger number of programs than those to which they apply. For example, while this will vary from specialty to specialty, for some primary care areas you might request applications from 20 programs. You might complete and submit only 15 of these, interviewing at 10, and ranking only seven or eight programs. Again, and very importantly, the above numbers will vary from specialty to specialty, and your faculty advisors should be helpful in guiding you to choose the appropriate number and types of programs based upon the competitiveness of each specialty and based upon your record.

SETTING YOUR PRIORITIES

Every applicant for residency training will have a different set of priorities and goals. We suggest that you strongly and carefully consider each program's academic environment and size in the process of selecting programs for application. Do not ignore the surrounding community or environment outside of the medical center in choosing programs as well. We urge you to request information from a large variety of programs so that you can better appreciate the multitude of options available to you.

Academic Environment

There is a wide variety of medical centers in which you may elect to train, ranging from academically oriented university centers, to university-affiliated or community-based programs, to county medical centers, to programs based at health maintenance organizations, and to training programs centered at Veterans Administration facilities. If you are seriously considering a career in academic medicine, you should concentrate on university-based programs or other programs where the faculty maintains full-time teaching and research commitments. You may want to be even more selective in seeking programs with particular strengths in a subspecialty of great interest to you (for example, adult cardiology), provided the basic residency curriculum provides a strong clinical foundation upon which you may build your academic career (e.g., broad-based training in general internal medicine).

Size

While some training programs will attempt to impress you with the large size of their house staff and the accompanying huge clinical load, others will emphasize the more personal nature and closer attention offered by their smaller department. We feel certain that you can receive strong training in either environment provided you are offered strong teaching with an appropriate clinical load. It may be useful for you to divide the total number of inpatient admissions by the number of house officers in each program to make a fair comparison of patient-to-resident ratios. While some interns will appreciate a very high patient load to build confidence, others prefer a somewhat smaller patient volume with additional time available for teaching, reading, and conferences. We suggest that you request literature on programs of all sizes and then select a program that offers the "happy-medium" of the above benefits to best suit your personal style and interests.

Surrounding Community

Do not underemphasize the importance of geographic location in selecting programs for application. If you are unhappy with the surrounding community for whatever reasons (e.g., size, crime rate, lack of cultural opportunities, distance from home, lack of employment opportunities for your spouse or significant other), then you will not be able to maximize your training experience to the extent that you would if you were personally more satisfied with your surroundings outside of the medical center. Remember that as a house officer in most specialties (especially during the first postgraduate year) you will have a limited amount of time to enjoy away from the hospital. You must, therefore, maximize your free time by selecting the environment that will best suit your needs and interests.

SEEKING ADVICE

There are four excellent sources of advice readily available to you as you select programs for internship application. These include the department chairman of the specialty of interest at your home institution, selected members of the faculty of the same department, senior medical students who are preparing for their own graduation and who have recently interviewed and experienced the "matching process," and house officers at your home institution who have chosen the same specialty and may be able to share their impressions from their own application process.

The department chairman is usually attuned to trends in the academic community and may offer a unique perspective on the strengths and weaknesses of individual programs. The chairman may also be informed about very recent or upcoming changes at institutions that you are considering. For example, current information on department chairman changes, faculty recruitment or losses, financial stability of the medical center, and clinical and research strengths may contribute toward your overall assessment. A counseling session with the chairman in the summer or early fall will not only help you focus upon appropriate programs to best suit your needs, but also provide the opportunity to discuss a chairman's letter of recommendation, which may be required by some programs.

You should seek a faculty advisor who has significant experience in guiding recent graduates through the internship selection process. Many departments will assign this responsibility to a member of the faculty who may serve as a counselor for all senior students interested in pursuing their particular area of postgraduate study. If this assigned person does not meet your specific needs, you should feel free to seek out a different advisor. Such advisors should be able to provide a list of the institutions where recent medical alumni are currently training. Do not be shy about calling these recent graduates with such candid questions as: "Would you choose the same program if given the opportunity to rank programs all over again?" and "How does your program compare with the training available at our medical school?"

Medical students in the class ahead of you are aware more frequently of the current status of training programs than either of the previously mentioned two resources. These students have visited the individual programs most recently and should be able to provide their perspectives on the various house staffs, the "esprit de corps" encountered with each visit, the competitiveness of each program, and other factors that you may not even have considered. Just before graduation you may want to organize a counseling session for all third-year students interested in a particular specialty and your senior student counterparts who have already matched with such programs and are preparing to leave for their internships.

House officers (especially interns) at your home institution may also be able to share their perspectives on programs that are of interest to you. Furthermore, they may have friends who are currently training at these centers and who may provide an "insider's view" into the training programs' strengths and weaknesses. We cannot overempha-

TABLE 4.1
Application Requirements and Planning Worksheet[a]

Program's Name Hospital	Program Director	Administrative Contact	Telephone Number	Application Deadline	Documents Required (DL, Letters (#?), USMLE, Transcript)	Program Interview Schedule (Specific Dates/Time Period)

[a]Adapted with permission from the UCLA School of Medicine, Office of Student Affairs.

size the importance of speaking with those who are currently enrolled within training programs.

After establishing your priorities with respect to academic strengths, size, location, and atmosphere in conjunction with the advice obtained from the preceding resources, you should request printed materials from the program directors as listed in the American Medical Association's computer AMA–FREIDA system by late summer or early fall. It is absolutely fine to send a neatly printed or typed postcard requesting this information. Formal letters are not necessary. If by August or September you are still uncertain about which specialty you would like to pursue after graduation, then we suggest you request literature from programs in all areas that you are considering seriously. This way, when you do commit yourself to a particular specialty by the late fall or early winter, you will have all of the application materials at hand and will not further delay the application process by having to wait for the requested forms. Most senior students request information from more programs than those to which they will actually apply. Given the constraints of time, distance, and finances, it is unusual for senior students to interview at more than 12–15 training programs. You may certainly elect to apply to many more programs initially, and can later narrow down your interview list to only those programs that you believe will truly best suit your needs and interests.

Once you have selected programs for application, you may choose to create an organized "table" of application requirements for each institution. We have included a sample format in Table 4.1. Each of the requirements of the application process will be addressed in some detail in the following chapter.

If possible, you may try keying in all relevant program addresses into a personal computer. This may enable you to print this list on "label sheets" for mailing, which would be greatly appreciated by the administrative assistants who will be preparing your letters. You might also be able to store this list on a diskette, which may be rerun every time you need to send documentation out to residency programs.

REFERENCES

1. American Medical Association. *Fellowship and Residency Electronic Interactive Database Access System (AMA–FREIDA),* American Medical Association, Chicago, 1998.
2. American Medical Association. *Directory of Graduate Medical Education Programs,* American Medical Association, Chicago, annual publication.

The Application

INTRODUCTION

The Universal Residency Application form was developed by the Association of American Medical Colleges (AAMC). It is distributed by the NRMP to its participants along with the NRMP Agreements. It is a generic application that may be reproduced and sent to many programs. This application form is designed to serve the needs of some programs rather than requiring applicants to fill out multiple applications requiring the same information in different formats. Some programs, however, may require you to complete their own application forms and will not accept the Universal Residency Application Form. It is anticipated at the time of publication that, for the 2000 Match, most students, however, will be able to use the Electronic Residency Application Service (ERAS), including students applying to Diagnostic Radiology, Emergency Medicine, Family Practice, Internal Medicine, OB/GYN, Orthopedics, Pediatrics, Surgery, Transitional Year Programs, and all

U.S. Army specialties, as well as some combined training programs (including Internal Medicine/Emergency Medicine, Internal Medicine/Family Practice, and Internal Medicine/Pediatrics). The Electronic Residency Application Service was developed by the Association of American Medical Colleges (AAMC) to facilitate the transmission via the Internet of residency applications, personal statements, letters of recommendation, Deans' Letters, transcripts, etc. from medical schools directly to Program Directors (1).

APPLICATION PHOTOGRAPH

Many applications for residency training will request a recent passport-sized photograph. A visit to a photographer by the end of the summer is in order. Be sure to dress appropriately and professionally for this photograph session. Casual photos on the beach, on camping trips, with pets, and in tee-shirts are not appropriate for this purpose. Your 2-inch by 2-inch photograph should be neatly mounted on page 3 of the Universal Residency Application Form. After receiving your Match results in the spring, most programs will request one or two additional photographs to prepare "identification sheets" of all incoming house staff. You may plan for this in advance by ordering extra photographs at the start of the application process.

APPLICATION PERSONAL STATEMENTS

While some programs may ask very specific questions of their applicants on supplemental materials, most will offer a less structured opportunity for you to share information about yourself and your interests. A wide variety of issues may be raised in your personal statement, including:

- Why you are selecting a particular specialty, or why you feel particularly well-suited for the specialty to which you are applying,

- What you're looking for in a residency training program,
- At this point in time, what long-range career plans are you considering after your residency training (e.g., academic medicine, private practice, public health, or Health Maintenance Organization),
- What are your impressive research accomplishments, publications, and/or awards that may have resulted in special recognition from the academic community,
- An autobiographical sketch summarizing your undergraduate years, family, etc., especially if they have had a strong impact on your career choice,
- Extracurricular activities, especially if they are not related to the study or practice of medicine (including hobbies, cultural interests, etc.),
- Unusual adventures, travel experiences, or outside interests,
- Any combination of the above.

You should not feel as though you need to discuss all of the items in the preceding list. Any combination may be appropriate, although, at the least, you should address why you are selecting a particular specialty, and what you're looking for in a residency training program. Do not feel as though you must include a detailed description of your upbringing or family history unless you would like to share with the reader how your earlier years may have contributed to your professional development.

Please do not fill a page repeating all of the information that will be included on your curriculum vitae, which should be submitted along with your other application materials. The personal statement does, however, provide an opportunity for you to expand upon items listed on your resumé that may be particularly worthy of highlighting. We also want to caution you against making your personal statement another AMCAS application essay, telling the reader all of the factors that stimulated you to pursue a career in medicine.

We feel it is also very important for you to communicate briefly some outside interests in your personal statement. In evaluating your credentials, a residency selection committee might appreciate knowing about your nonacademic extracurricular activities, including sports, travel, foreign languages, film, theater, reading, music, and dancing. For example, if you have had an unusual hiking adventure in the Himalayan Mountains or have gone bungee-jumping over the Zambezi River, then share this information in your personal statement. A two- to three-sentence description of these outside interests usually placed at the end of your personal statement may serve as a springboard for a relaxing conversation with an interviewer who may share similar interests.

Your personal statement should be clear, concise, and articulate. This statement need not have a theme nor be particularly eccentric or flashy. While we encourage creativity, we caution you that extremely unusual personal statements run the risk of being viewed negatively by some readers. Avoid nonprofessional comments such as "Ever since I began carving the Thanksgiving turkey at age 12, I knew that I wanted to be a surgeon" or "I knew I wanted to pursue a career in obstetrics at age 10 when I watched my pet beagle give birth to a litter of puppies."

We recommend that you condense your thoughts into no more than 1–1½ typed pages, as longer personal statements may not be read in their entirety by interviewers or by application screeners. Your essay should be neatly typed within the space provided on page 1 of the Universal Residency Application Form, or it may be typed separately and attached to your application. Please don't use excessively tiny print just to squeeze it onto one page, and no doodling or artwork in the margins! Be sure that your name is typed on your personal statement to avoid any filing confusion.

The final draft of your personal statement should be proofread carefully for typographical, grammatical, and spelling errors. All typing should be neatly and professionally prepared with appropriate margins and spacing. We encourage you to ask your faculty advisor to review your essay. (Some faculty members may wish to have a copy of your personal statement in addition to your curriculum vitae before composing a letter of recommendation.) Remember, this is your opportunity to shine on paper. As an applicant, if you don't present yourself neatly and articulately when you have a lot of time to prepare your personal statement, what will your admission and progress notes be like when you're running around, busy on call? If you're uncomfortable with your writing skills, please be sure to have others review your personal statement before you send it.

LETTERS OF RECOMMENDATION

All applicants for residency training will require a Dean's letter of recommendation. Generally, your Dean of Student Affairs, or his or her designee, will complete a letter that summarizes your background, your performance in the basic sciences, your performance clinically (including comments from each of your core clerkships), and a bit about your extracurricular interests and/or activities. Please note that there is a national policy that Dean's letters are not mailed out until November 1 of each year.

In addition, many applications will require a letter from a department chairperson (or his or her designee) in addition to two or three other letters of recommendation. Unless you feel that many different members of the faculty have a significantly different perspective on your performance, it will probably not be in your best interest to solicit more letters of recommendation than those requested by each program. Remember, a *thicker* application file does *not* necessarily make for a stronger file, so please don't go overboard soliciting extra letters! At the same time, you should not feel that all letters of recommendation must come solely from faculty members within the specialty to which you are applying. In addition to your Dean's letter and Chairman's letter, a reasonable approach would be to solicit three additional letters of recommendation with at least one or two of these letters from members of the faculty within your specialty of interest. A letter from a faculty member in the Department of Internal Medicine is often helpful because Internal Medicine is universally considered to be a taxing and rigorous third-year rotation. It may also be to your advantage to solicit your letters from more senior members of the faculty who may be known by others within their specialties at the regional and national level. *The greatest priority, however, in selecting faculty to write on your behalf is to choose faculty members who know you best.* Please do not ask someone to write for you if you do not feel that the person will be able to communicate about a working relationship close enough to assess your abilities accurately.

Once you have selected faculty members to submit letters on your behalf, you should schedule an appointment to meet with each of these people early in the application process (i.e., by September or October). It is polite and appropriate to ask each person if he or she believes that your abilities are known well enough to submit a positive letter of recommendation on your behalf. If so, you should discuss your career goals and, at the same time, solicit advice about programs to which you should apply (see Chapter 4).

Each faculty member who agrees to write a letter of recommendation for you should receive an up-to-date curriculum vitae and a copy of your personal statement. Most faculty members will also have access to your academic records in the Dean's office should they require additional information on your performance on other services or in the basic sciences.

You must plan ahead in soliciting letters of recommendation with at least several weeks of advance notice to each faculty member before requesting that your letters be mailed to the programs to which you are applying. Many programs will not even screen your application file, nor invite you for an interview until your application is complete (including receipt of all letters of recommendation). Remember that faculty members may take vacation during the summer or early fall months and may be unavailable to you for solicitation of letters. To avoid some of these delays, you should solicit your references as early as possible at the start of your senior year. Some students have even requested recommendations as early as their junior year as they finish a clerkship with the faculty member in question (that is, provided they have performed well on the service and have had significant exposure to the attending involved).

In addition to an up-to-date curriculum vitae, you should provide the faculty member's administrative assistant with a neatly prepared typewritten list of the names and addresses of the program directors to whom you would like your references sent. This will usually be the same list that you will submit to the Dean of Student Affairs Office (see Figure 5.1). A set of mailing labels for the administrative staff within the Student Affairs office, as well as for the assistants who will be mailing out your letters, would be greatly appreciated. Within several weeks after meeting with each attending, you may want to call each assistant to make sure that your letters are being prepared for mailing.

THE CURRICULUM VITAE

There are many different styles and formats that you may use for preparing your curriculum vitae. Regardless of the format selected, your resumé should provide for the reader a neat, concise summary of your academic and extracurricular activities, in addition to some basic biographical data. In most instances, your curriculum vitae should be condensed into one typewritten page and may be attached to your application form. Do not try to include long distracting explanations of your employment, extracurricular activities, and

Student's Name _____

Specialty(ies) Applying In: _____

Name & Address of Hospital   Program Director

1. _____   _____
   _____
   _____
   _____

2. _____   _____
   _____
   _____
   _____

3. _____   _____
   _____
   _____
   _____

4. _____   _____
   _____
   _____
   _____

5. _____   _____
   _____
   _____
   _____

6. _____   _____
   _____
   _____
   _____

Figure 5.1. Hospital Address List for Dean's Letter. Adapted with permission from the UCLA School of Medicine, Office of Student Affairs.

	Date Application to Be Sent or Already Sent
Dept. of Specialty	
_____	_____
_____	_____
_____	_____
_____	_____
_____	_____

JOHN DOE
CURRICULUM VITAE

Home Address & Telephone
123 Main Street
Apartment A
Hometown, USA 00000
(Area Code)—Telephone #

Biographical Data
Date of Birth:
Place of Birth:
Social Security #:
Marital Status: (optional)

Education

1996–2000 —Medical School, City, and State
          —MD anticipated in May, 2000
1992–1996 —Undergraduate Institution, City and State
          —Degree earned, major (and Greek honors if applicable)

Honors and Awards

"Date   —Name of Honor and Award, followed by
          Name of School"

Examples:
1998   —Medical Alumni Scholarship,
          Name of Medical School
1996   —Phi Beta Kappa, Name of College

Certification

United States Medical Licensing Examination,
    Step I: Month, Year—Percentile (or Passed)
United States Medical Licensing Examination,
    Step II: Month, Year—Pending

Research Experience

"Date—Title of Investigation, Supervisor, location"

Example: 1999—Investigation of "(title of research project)"
        under _____ MD,
        Dept. of _____, Name of Medical School

Publications

(Use standard reference format)

Extracurricular Activities and Employment

"Date—One-line summary of each activity and/or job"

Memberships

1996–1999 —American Medical Student's Association

Outside Interests _____, _____, _____, _____.

Figure 5.2. Sample curriculum vitae.

research involvement. You will have opportunities to expand upon the information listed on your curriculum vitae in your personal statement and, perhaps, during your interview. We have included a "sample format" (Figure 5.2) to assist you in the preparation of your resumé. Once again, you may choose among many different formats as long as your curriculum vitae is neat, well-organized, and complete.

A note of caution regarding the "home address" used on your curriculum vitae. While you may choose to put your medical school mailbox number on your resumé, be certain that you will be able to check this mailing address throughout the fall and winter months to receive communication from the programs to which you are applying. If you are planning to be away from your home institution for extramural electives or travel, you must be certain that your mail is appropriately screened and forwarded if necessary. To avoid this potential confusion, you may want to place only your permanent mailing address on your curriculum vitae.

Many students inquire as to whether their United States Medical Licensing Examination (USMLE) scores should be included on their resumé. You may choose to document the dates (month and year) when you took these examinations and should then state whether you have received passing scores. Although you may not have your scores from Step II of the USMLE before mailing out your applications, you may still state the date of the examination on your curriculum vitae. If you did particularly well on any of the above exams, you may want to state your scores as follows:

Board Certification:

USMLE, Step I—Month/Year—Score or Percentile
USMLE, Step II—Month/Year—Score or Percentile

Some medical students will be elected to the Alpha Omega Alpha (AOA) Honor Medical Society during the fall of their senior year after their curriculum vitae and applications have been mailed out. If this is the case, you should ensure that all programs are updated immediately on the change in status of your application. This may be accomplished by having your Dean of Medical Student Affairs office write to all of the programs to which you have applied, or by writing personally to notify them of your election.

TRANSCRIPTS

Most applications for residency training will require a copy of your medical school transcript and, on occasion, you may have to submit transcripts from undergraduate and other graduate education. You should request mailing of these transcripts by the early fall by providing your medical school Registrar's office with a neatly prepared typewritten list of the names and addresses of the program directors to whom you would like your transcript sent. Alternatively, many schools will automatically send out your transcript along with your Dean's letter of recommendation.

ADDITIONAL TIPS FOR YOUR APPLICATION

Upon registering with the National Resident Matching Program, you will be assigned an "NRMP Number." Each training program, in turn, has its own NRMP Number, which is published in the NRMP Directory in the spring of each year. You will be asked to record your number on page 3 of the Universal Residency Application Form. It is particularly important that you notify all programs to which you have applied of your NRMP number. Please be sure not to misplace your number!

Much of the information requested on the Universal

Residency Application Form will also be addressed in your personal statement or in your curriculum vitae. It is inappropriate for you to write "see C.V." in every space. Rather, you should try to answer the questions individually, even if you must abbreviate.

Some lines of questioning on application materials may not apply to you specifically. For example, not every applicant has conducted research, yet many forms will provide space for you to summarize your research activities and publications. Do not worry about leaving these sections blank if you have no research experience and have not published.

Photographs most often are optional. If you do choose to include a photo (and most applicants do), please don't send a scary one! Once again, presenting yourself neatly and professionally is the theme.

PHOTOCOPY YOUR APPLICATION

It is generally a good idea to copy all application materials before mailing them. It will be useful to review your answers to the essay questions on your application forms before each interview. Remember to pack these photocopies (along with the literature sent by each training program, which describes each program's curriculum) when you leave on your interview trip.

REFERENCES

1. *NRMP Handbook for Students,* National Resident Matching Program, Washington, D.C. 1998.

Interviewing

SCHEDULING TIPS

Most fourth-year medical students should schedule a 1-month block of time between November and February for interviewing. Early planning is essential as you begin the internship interviewing process. You will find that many programs will not even schedule appointments until all of your application materials (including all references and Dean's letter) are received. Therefore, if you are planning to interview in November, you may need to encourage faculty members politely to mail their letters of recommendation promptly. Depending on the competitiveness of the specialty and the individual programs involved, many residency selection committees will prescreen their applications and offer interviews on an invitation basis only. Once invited, you will find some programs to be less flexible than others with the actual dates available for interviewing. Some institutions will offer interviews throughout the fall and winter on selected days of the week only (for example, every Tuesday and Thursday), whereas others will offer an even more limited selection of interview dates (e.g., 1 or 2 days per month from November through January or February). It will be a significant advantage for you to plan ahead in scheduling your interviews to meet the constraints of the programs for which you are most interested. Alternative-day interviews or special considerations requested on your behalf may be viewed negatively by the program and may be less than an ideal visit for you. Special requests require busy faculty to schedule interviews on days that they are slated to be doing something else. Programs where particular days are established for interviewing generally include an orientation from the program director or chairman, special tours arranged by house officers, interviews by scheduled faculty, and possibly lunch or another less intense opportunity to see the program. On alternative interview days you will be fortunate if you see the facility and have a brief faculty interview. Avoid getting "closed out" of interviews because other candidates have filled all available interview positions for a given date. Remember that there are only a limited number of interviewers available on any given date at any given program. We recommend that you systematically list all of the programs to which you have been invited for interviews along with the available days for interviewing at each center. Such scheduling should begin by October or November regardless of whether you are planning to complete your interviews in the late fall or winter. It is probably wise to schedule your first interviews at programs of "lesser desirability," because you will certainly become more polished and more comfortable with interviewing with added experience. You should also try to schedule at least one full day at each program facility. If, after scheduling an interview appointment, you decide that you would like to decline the interview invitation, *please* call the program to cancel so that other students may be accommodated. Please do not be a "no show" without canceling, as this reflects very poorly on you and your school!

TIPS FOR TRAVEL ARRANGEMENTS

Travel expenses will accumulate rapidly if you choose to interview at many centers far from your home city. Students in need of funds for the interview process should check with the financial aid office of their medical schools to see if any assistance is available. We can recommend several ways to help you minimize the costs of lodging and travel.

Before leaving home, you should consult your medical school Alumni Directory for the names, addresses, and phone numbers of alumni residing in the cities where you will be visiting. Not only may such alumni provide an "insider's view" into the training programs or institutions that you will be visiting, but you may be offered overnight accommodations at their homes to help defray costs. Administrative personnel at training programs may also be able to recommend inexpensive overnight accommodations that will be convenient to the medical center. Some programs may have arranged for a discount rate for applicants staying at particular hotels and motels. In other centers, on-call quarters may be available for overnight stay.

The National Organization of Student Representatives has established a National Housing Bureau to help medical students cut costs while interviewing. For each medical school to participate in this program there must be at least 10 students at each school who volunteer their homes to host students who are interviewing in their city. You may inquire with the Dean of Student Affairs Office as to whether your medical school is participating in this program. The National Organization of Student Representatives is coordinated by the Association of American Medical Colleges [(202) 828-0682].

For those applying to early match specialties, some of the independent matching programs provide a reference to a national travel agency that has built a database of lodging, car rental, and other information (provided by the training programs) for each interview city. This agency also has negotiated discounts for coach and supersaver airfares with major carriers for prospective resident trainees. If interested, please request additional information from the individual matching programs as listed in Chapter 3.

Punctuality is extremely important and all travel arrangements should take into account unanticipated delays. If you are traveling long distances and will be required to arrive at the institution in the early morning, we suggest that you arrive the evening before your interview to familiarize yourself with the institution and to assure that you are on time.

PREPARATION TIPS

We strongly recommend that you participate in "practice interviews" with a member of the faculty at your home institution. Not only may "rehearsals" help lessen your anxieties, but you may also be confronted with several unanticipated questions for which you will appreciate the extra time to prepare clear, well thought-out responses.

You should receive written or telephone confirmation of all of your appointments before you embark on your interview trip. If you do not, we recommend that you call the interview coordinators at the Offices of Graduate Medical Education at each institution to avoid any miscommunication. Many programs request phone confirmation the day before your interview.

It goes without saying that you should arrive on time. Also, you will want to bring an adequate supply of interview outfits to present yourself in a neat and professional manner. Regardless of how you are accustomed to dressing at home, at work, or at school, you do not want to be remembered by your interviewers for what you were wearing. Do not show up with blue hair, sneakers, and tennis shorts, even if they have an alligator on them! Although we make light of this topic with these examples, accessories should be in good taste and would not include a lucky rabbit's foot on a chain or worry beads.

It's very important to arrive well-prepared! Be sure to pack all printed materials received from each program before you leave home on your interview trip. It is essential for you to review this literature on the evening or morning just before your visit. You should approach each interview day with at least a basic understanding of the information presented in these printed materials to maximize your experience at each center. This approach will minimize the chances of asking questions that are already clearly answered in the program's brochure and will provide you with the opportunity to clarify areas of uncertainty. Arriving with some basic understanding of the institution and training program will also help you appear more interested, well-versed, and very organized. Please make your questions pertinent and well-focused.

THE IMPORTANCE OF THE INTERVIEW

The interview provides the applicant with very useful information about the esprit de corps of the house staff and "milieu of the institution" (1). At the same time, the interview provides the faculty with a valuable glimpse of the applicant's personality and other noncognitive factors, which may be predictive of the student's performance in a residency training program (2).

Please keep in mind that in addition to answering your questions about their program, interviewers are seeking to assess your maturity, commitment to hard work, and compatibility with the program.

In the mid-1980s Wagoner, Suriano, and Stoner reviewed extensively the factors used by program directors to select residents (3). Their results were consistent with an earlier study (4) indicating that the interview was considered to be the most important selection criterion by greater than 200 program directors polled in multiple specialties. The applicant's "compatibility with the program," maturity, and commitment to hard work were found to be important variables determined by the interview. However, with recent trends toward greater competition for some postgraduate training positions, program directors are now relying quite heavily on academic performance in screening applicants before even granting an interview. Furthermore, the focus of individual interviews will likely now reflect recent changes in graduate medical education, including the emphasis on generalism, the increase in managed care, and other trends in academic medicine.

TIPS FOR THE INTERVIEW

Your interviewers will be trying to assess your maturity, articulateness, professionalism, enthusiasm, interests, and responsibility. A mild degree of nervousness is not unusual and will most often be discounted by your interviewer. Try to remain calm and at ease with yourself without putting on false airs. The great majority of interviews will not be high-pressured interrogations but will provide the opportunity for a pleasant and mutually rewarding exchange of information. It is imperative to have your thoughts on your professional goals and choice of specialty organized beforehand. On rare occasions, you may be asked a factual question or asked to present a case for your interviewer (be prepared with a brief and interesting case history just in case).

Be sure to ask intelligent questions about the training program, as a lack of inquiry may be falsely interpreted as disinterest. You may want to have several questions in mind even before you begin your interview. Some examples include:

1. What are the greatest strengths and weaknesses of this program? (This is a vastly overused question and often conveys to the interviewer that you have given no thought to the characteristics of their particular institution. However, if you communicate your understanding of the program, this question can be asked in the context of subspecialties covered or deficient, research opportunities, house staff morale, and teaching, to name a few.)

2. What paths have most of your recent graduates taken following completion of their training?

3. What are you looking for in a candidate and how might I fit into your program?

4. Do you feel that the volume of patients seen on both the inpatient and outpatient services provides an appropriate patient load per house officer?

5. Is there a pyramid system for promotion in your program?

6. What are the details of the fringe benefit package for house officers (for example, health and dental insurance for the house officers and their families)?

7. What are the major research interests within the department?

8. From what medical schools have your current residents graduated?

9. Are your house officers encouraged and funded to attend a continuing medical education course or conference during each academic year?

10. Can you describe the structure of your continuity clinics, and the extent to which the residents are excused from their other responsibilities to attend?

11. How did your residents do on this year's in-service examination?

12. What major changes are anticipated in the department and/or medical center and in what direction is the program headed?

13. How would you assess the level of camaraderie and "esprit de corps" among the house staff? (Ask this question of both the faculty and house staff.)

14. What is the relationship between private admitting physicians and the house officers, and do the house officers have enough independence in the management of the private patients?
15. What elective opportunities are available to your house officers?
16. How would you describe the didactic teaching program?
17. How have your residents done on their Board-certifying examinations?
18. When alone with the house staff, be sure to ask them if they would choose this program if they had to make the selection all over again.
19. Ask the house staff if the faculty and administration are receptive to their suggestions versus being dictatorial.
20. Ask the house staff about their outside interests. Do they have time to enjoy themselves outside of work? (This is of critical importance in assessing lifestyle issues and your compatibility with the program and its people.)
21. Ask the house staff about the adequacy of the hospital's ancillary services, as this may affect your available time for reading and learning.
22. What changes do you anticipate in the program over the next 5 years?
23. Ask the program director if the program's recent graduates describe any inadequacies in preparing them for clinical practice.
24. Ask the program director what he or she would change if there was one thing to be changed about the training program.
25. Does your program have a teaching curriculum in ethics?
26. How is current health care reform affecting this medical center? (This has become increasingly important, and we feel that this question should be addressed at least once during each program visit.)

To prepare for your interviews, we suggest that you ask the following questions of yourself before your first interview. Develop your best possible answers to these questions even if you are uncertain. You should realize that everybody expects you to be goal oriented but not committed to these answers, and your philosophy should reflect an openness to change based upon your residency experiences. Typical questions asked by interviewers include:

1. What are your interests outside of medicine?
2. What are your plans after residency?
3. Where do you see yourself in 10 years?
4. What are you looking for in a training program?
5. How do you feel about working with private physicians, and have you had any such experience?
6. Why have you chosen this particular specialty?
7. What aspects of this particular training program or specialty are particularly attractive to you? . . . or are of particular concern to you?
8. How have you been employed during the past 5 years, and what have you learned from these jobs or experiences?
9. What are your hobbies?
10. What books have you read recently?
11. Do you prefer any specific geographic location, and why?
12. Who recommended our program to you?
13. What are your major strengths? . . . and weaknesses?
14. What questions do you have for us about this residency training program?
15. Please discuss the future of medicine and its effects on individual physicians and your career plans.
16. In which direction do you see this specialty heading in the next 10 years, and how can you contribute to this field?
17. Why should I choose you over one of your classmates?
18. What would you do if you did not obtain a residency position for next year?
19. Tell me about yourself.

TURNOFFS

Several factors will assuredly turn off your interviewers from the start, including a sloppy personal appearance, poor manners, and lack of maturity. Make sure you arrive promptly for your interview; if you are unavoidably delayed, you should call ahead and provide a good explanation for your tardiness. Do not be argumentative with the administrative personnel or anyone else involved in the matching process. Other turnoffs include overaggressive, overbearing behavior, strong prejudices, narrow interests, and condemnation of other specialties. Do not look at your watch repetitively throughout the interview. Do not emphasize "connections" or influential individuals and be prepared to accept constructive criticism.

TIPS ON ASSESSING THE PROGRAM AND COMMUNITY

It will be in your best interest to spend as much time as possible at any given institution to assess the house staff and faculty both formally and informally. Take advantage of opportunities to revisit the wards and clinics to discuss the program with the house staff even after your official interviewing has been completed. Assess the level of satisfaction of the current residents and their sense of camaraderie and support. Ask them candidly whether they would choose the same training program if given the opportunity to decide all over again. Be sure to get the name and telephone number of at least one house officer at every program whom you may contact at a later date with additional questions. After the formal interview activities, you might want to roam around the wards or clinics to meet and talk with as many of the residents as possible. No brochure really tells you what the house staff think of the program.

With the rapid changes in health care today, it's important for you to carefully assess the patient base and financial stability of each medical center involved in the program. *This is absolutely critical!*

It is equally important to assess the community surrounding the medical center. Make sure you leave with a solid understanding of the cost of living, areas in which the house staff currently reside, employment opportunities for your spouse or significant other, and cultural and recreational activities.

All of your impressions should be recorded soon after leaving each training program. We assure you that the details of each center will soon be forgotten or confused if not committed to paper in an organized fashion. List the important "positives" and "negatives" in order of priority, including your impressions of the house staff, faculty, "esprit de corps," curriculum, geographic location, physical plant, and benefits. Be sure to record any questions that might be answered with a follow-up telephone call or letter to the program director or chief resident. Alternatively, you might consider completion of the "Residency Program Summary Sheet" (Fig. 6.1), which should be completed on the same day or night after leaving your interview.

Once you have finished the interview process, you may want to consider revisiting a program if you have enough time, finances, and energy. Remember that your initial impressions may be based on quite subjective and uncontrollable circumstances and may be interpreted differently on a repeat visit (e.g., was your tour guide irritable and somewhat unfriendly after an exhausting and difficult night on call?). Most programs would be delighted to have you visit them again in either an informal or formal fashion.

Thank you letters after your interviews are appropriate yet certainly not mandatory. You may want to take the opportunity to express your appreciation for the time given to you; and if you are still honestly excited about a training program, explain very briefly your continuing interest. Such letters also provide opportunities to include updated information about yourself.

Residency Program Summary Sheet

Program _____

Interview Date _____

Name(s) of Interviewer(s) _____

I. Current House Staff
    —Size_____
    —Esprit de Corps _____
    —Happiness _____
    —Other Comments _____
    _____
    _____

II. Workload
     —Call Schedule _____
     —Patient Volume _____
     —Level of Independence _____
     —Time to Read _____
     —Time to Attend Conferences _____
     —Other Comments _____

III. Faculty
      —Availability of Attending Staff _____
      —Availability of Subspecialty Coverage _____
      —Preceptors in Clinic? On Wards? _____
      —Percentage of Full-time Teaching Faculty _____

IV. Education
     —Who does the teaching (H.S., Faculty, Fellows)? ___
     —Teaching Conferences and Education Curriculum __
       (Grand Rounds, Clinical Conferences, House Staff
       Lectures) _____
     —House Officer Curriculum Requirements _____

Figure 6.1.

    (required rotations vs. selectives vs. electives) ___
    —What have the graduates gone on to do? _____
    (Fellowships, Practice, HMO, etc.) _____

  V. Medical Center
    —Type of hospital _____
    (Community vs. University vs. HMO) _____
    —Financial Stability_____
    —Ancillary Services _____
    (incl. Venipuncture, Transport) _____
    —Laboratory Services _____
    —Patient Information _____
    —Primary Care vs. Tertiary _____
    —Social and Socioeconomic Backgrounds _____

  VI. Compensation
    —Annual Salary _____
    —Vacation Leave _____
    —Educational Leave (conferences, etc.) _____
    —Maternity and Sick Leave _____

 VII. Community
    —Strengths _____
    —Weaknesses _____

VIII. Overall Impressions

_____

_____

_____

_____

_____

_____

_____

Figure 6.1.—*continued*

REFERENCES

1. Komives E, Weiss S, Rosa R. The applicant interview as a predictor of resident performance. *J Med Educ* 1984; 59:425–426.
2. Gong H Jr, Parker N, Apgar F, Shank C. Influence of the interview on ranking in the residency selection process. *Med Educ* 1984; 18:366–369.
3. Wagoner N, Suriano J, Stoner J. Factors used by program directors to select residents. *J Med Educ* 1986; 61:10–21.
4. Wagoner N, Gray G. Report on a survey of program directors regarding selection factors in graduate medical education. *J Med Educ* 1979; 54:445–452.

Ranking

INTRODUCTION

All applicants and residency training programs will enter their rank lists via the World Wide Web by mid-February of each year. While applicants will have a different set of priorities as they assess programs to establish their own rank lists, *we suggest that your number one priority be a strong training experience in an environment where you can be happy and thrive!* Be sure that you like the "personalities" of all programs that you are ranking. In comparing institutions, you might be torn by many factors, including the size of the programs, the academic reputations, how graduates fare on board certification exams, and what percentage of the graduates pursue careers in academic medicine versus private practice. All of these aspects will collectively create a "gestalt impression" as to whether you would like to train in a particular setting. In establishing such priorities for yourself, do not underestimate the importance of personal happiness for you and your family.

After an interview day, some programs will just feel right to you, and you may not be able to articulate the reasons for this attraction or sense of appeal. Do not ignore this feeling; in fact, consider it to be one of *critical* importance throughout the ranking process. When you respond to this "gut feeling," be sure to review the information tabulated on your "Residency Program Summary Sheet" (see Fig. 6.1) to be certain that you understand the specifics of each program that you are considering. To allay uncertainties, you may want to revisit programs that you are considering ranking. If this is economically impossible or infeasible, consider a phone call to the residency program director, current chief resident, or a current house officer to address lingering doubts or concerns.

Over the years, we have certainly shared the anxieties of so many of our own advisees as they have sorted out the ranking process. While we appreciate that it's easier said than done, we'd like to urge you to maintain your perspective on the process, and hope that the following analogy will be helpful to you in maintaining your perspective:

In some ways, the process of choosing a residency program is like choosing dessert. When making your choice for this next "course" in your education, try not to lose your perspective. For most students who are wrestling with how to sort out the order of their top couple of choices, it's important to remember that the choice is not between apple pie and arsenic. Instead, it's more likely that you're choosing between apple pie and an ice cream sundae. Aspects of one program may be "sweeter" to you than aspects of other programs, and classmates may or may not share the same "tastes" or impressions of each program. Once you feel comfortable that you can receive fine training at each of your top choices (keeping in mind that every program has different strengths as well as weaknesses, and that there's always room for improvement at every program), your decision becomes a visceral one. Remember to "trust your heart!"

In Chapter 6 we emphasized the importance of assessing the details of each program. After having looked at the details of each "tree," take a step backward and "take in the whole forest." We can't emphasize enough how important it is for you to ask yourself over and over again the following questions about each program:

- How did I feel there?
- Do I think I could fit in?
- Would I like to be part of that group of people?

Think about Match Day and picture yourself ripping open your Match results and seeing Program "X" written on your Match slip. Try to register this emotional response and your anticipated level of excitement and factor these in when you make up your final rank order list.

We have some other general tips for you to consider before establishing your rank list. Ranking a program is a commitment to train at that program if a match results. If you have any doubts, do not rank the program. It is far better for you not to match than to match at a program or in a city about which you have strong negative feelings. If you are pursuing a competitive field, your competitiveness needs to be discussed with your advisors. In this case, it is wise to have other options on your rank list, including other less competitive specialties. If you already know what subspecialty you would like to pursue after your residency, consider training programs with academically strong divisions in this subspecialty to provide you with both good teaching in this area and effective references for your subsequent fellowship training. If you are undecided as to whether you would like to pursue a career in academic medicine, then lean toward more academic programs to maximize your options upon graduation. If you are certain that you are aiming for a career in private practice and are still somewhat undecided between two programs, then consider geographic location as an important factor to establish hospital ties. Additionally, do not be shy about aiming high by including very competitive programs at the top of your rank list. It should *not* be important to you how far down your match list you go before matching. It is a greater priority to maximize your training opportunities and to allow the computer to match your preferences with those of the programs. At the same time, be sure not to overestimate yourself. Regardless of how comfortable you may be that you will match at your number one choice, it would be prudent to include additional programs on your list (but again, only if you feel as though you would enjoy training in these other programs). You will not be penalized for including additional listings.

Confidentiality of rank lists must be maintained by applicants and by residency program directors. It is inappropriate for applicants to solicit information on their rank position from the institutions to which they have applied. Similarly, residency program directors should not pressure applicants to accept contracts for appointment before Match Day. All too frequently, students are shocked and disappointed on Match Day after having been told by program directors that they would be the program's number one choice. Both applicants and residency program directors have the right to change their rank lists before the final deadline for submission to the NRMP.

Match Day

INTRODUCTION

Match Day for the NRMP typically occurs in the middle of March and is the culmination of the long process of residency selection. While match results have traditionally been released at each school by the Dean of Student Affairs Office, independent applicants and U.S. students may access their match results on the NRMP Web Page and via the NRMP Voice Response System, utilizing their NRMP codes and PIN codes. Many institutions will plan a celebration in conjunction with Match Day activities. It is appropriate for you to bring your spouse or significant other to provide support and to share your excitement as you open your match envelope.

The great majority of U.S. seniors will match with one of their top choices. In fact, more than 50% of U.S. seniors in the 1998 Match obtained their first choices. Figure 8.1 summa-

U.S. Seniors
1998 Match

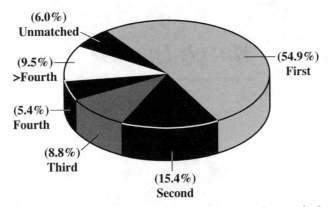

(6.0%) Unmatched

(9.5%) >Fourth

(5.4%) Fourth

(8.8%) Third

(15.4%) Second

(54.9%) First

Figure 8.1. Percentage of United States seniors who matched to their first, second, third, fourth, fifth or lower ranked programs in the NRMP 1998 Match. Adapted with permission from the National Resident Matching Program (1).

rizes the data of U.S. seniors in 1998 who matched to their first, second, third, fourth, fifth or lower ranked programs.

The unmatched applicant faces significant emotional turmoil. At the time of publication, the NRMP began initiating a number of alterations for the scheduling of "Match Week," but it is likely that for the 2000 Match, unmatched U.S. seniors will be notified of their predicament by their Student Affairs Office at least 48 hours before the announcement of match results later in the week. Such students will meet with their Deans of Student Affairs to discuss alternative options for training from a list of programs with unfilled positions. Their respective department chairmen will frequently intervene and help solicit placement with their colleagues at unfilled institutions. Please note that there are very *strict* rules about when this "Scramble

Process" may begin—i.e., the time when negotiations may begin to fill unfilled positions. Each year, many unmatched students end up doing far better than they would have, given the programs on their original rank list. Many programs that go unfilled are excellent places to train. The vast majority of unmatched students will be placed in positions within 48 hours, but not all can be placed in their first choice of specialty. A summary of the percentage of United States students who chose to rank only one type of specialty and went unmatched in 1998 is summarized in Figure 8.2 (1).

Unmatched "independent applicants" may also solicit placement in unfilled programs by directly contacting the residency program directors at those institutions.

As a reminder, applicants and hospitals matched through the NRMP are contractually bound to one another —i.e., programs are committed to offer an official appointment to each matched applicant who has met their prerequisites and institutional employment conditions, and applicants are committed to enter the positions into which they have been matched (2). Each matched applicant is obligated to sign a contract letter or letter of appointment, which will be sent by the training institution, usually within 1 month of Match Day.

INDEPENDENT MATCHING PROGRAMS

Match results will be released in January or February for independent Matching Programs in Neurological Surgery, Neurology, Ophthalmology, and Otolaryngology, and in April for programs in Plastic Surgery. These independent matching programs provide "vacancy line recordings" for most specialties and all fellowships so that programs have an easy way of advertising vacancies and applicants may find them quickly. For more detailed information, call the Vacancy Line Recording at (415) 447-0350 and follow the voicemail in-

Figure 8.2
U.S. Seniors Who Ranked Only One Type of Specialty and Who Went Unmatched in 1998 *

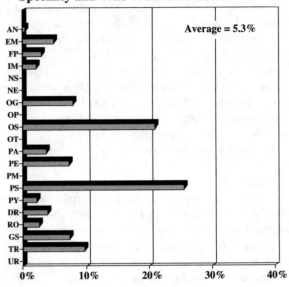

All Choices

Key:	
AN = Anesthesiology	**PA** = Pathology
EM = Emergency Medicine	**PE** = Pediatrics
FP = Family Practice	**PM** = Phys Medicine & Rehab
IM = Internal Medicine	**PS** = Plastic Surgery
NS = Neurological Surgery	**PY** = Psychiatry
NE = Neurology	**DR** = Diagnostic Radiology
OG = Obstetrics-Gynecology	**RO** = Radiation-Oncology
OP = Ophthalmology	**GS** = General Surgery
OS = Orthopedic Surgery	**TR** = Transitional
OT = Otolaryngology	**UR** = Urology

Figure 8.2. NRMP data on United States medical students who chose to rank only one type of specialty who went unmatched in 1998 by specialty. Adapted with permission from National Resident Matching Program (2).
* These statistics do not include data from the Independent Matching Programs

TABLE 8.1
Matches for Independent Matching Programs

	Neurol-ogy	Neuro-surgery	Ophthal-mology	Otolaryn-gology	Urology
Average Number of Applications	17	31	30	37	30
Average Number of Interviews	4.4	10.0	7.6	8.1	9.9
Percentage of U.S. Seniors who Matched	96%	71%	91%	72%	73%
Percentage of U.S. Graduates who Matched	52%	29%	59%	43%	40%
Percentage of FMGs who Matched	36%	15%	28%	20%	5%

Table 8.1. Data from selected independent matching programs from 1998 Match. Adapted with permission from Neurology Matching Program, Neurological Surgery Matching Program, Ophthalmology Matching Program, Otolaryngology Matching Program (3) and Urology Matching Program (4).

structions. Vacancy listings for these programs and related Fellowships may also be accessed via the following web site: www.SFMATCH.org. Please note that given the "Two Tier Match" in Neurology (see Table 1.1), unfilled positions are frozen and may be offered again in the subsequent match year.

Statistics from selected independent matching programs from the 1998 Match are summarized in Table 8.1.

REFERENCES

1. *NRMP Data—March, 1998,* National Resident Matching Program, Washington, DC, 1998.
2. *NRMP Handbook for Students,* National Resident Matching Program, Washington, D.C., 1998.
3. Data from various independent matching programs, San Francisco, California, 1998. (Data from August Colenbrander, M.D.)
4. Data from AUA Urology Matching Program, Houston, Texas, 1998.

Tips for the International Medical Graduate

INTRODUCTION

An international medical graduate (IMG) is defined by the Educational Commission for Foreign Medical Graduates (ECFMG) as a physician who graduated from a medical school located outside of the United States, Canada, and Puerto Rico, regardless of citizenship status.

The ECFMG coordinates the eligibility process for international graduates to commence residency or fellowship training in programs accredited by the Accreditation Council for Graduate Medical Education (ACGME). According to the regulations of the ACGME, all graduates of foreign medical schools must hold a valid ECFMG Certificate to be eligible to participate in ACGME-accredited programs of graduate medical education. Since requirements for training may change periodically, it is critical that before applying to post-graduate programs, you acquire a copy of this year's *Information Booklet-ECFMG Certification* which includes some applications and information on the USMLE Step 1 and Step 2 Exams, the ECFMG English Test, and the relatively recently introduced ECFMG Clinical Skills Assessment (CSA), which includes an assessment of spoken English proficiency. This reference will provide a detailed explanation of testing requirements, as well as specific information on preparing for all examinations. You may request copies from:

> Educational Commission for Foreign Medical Graduates
> 3624 Market Street, 4th Floor
> Philadelphia, Pennsylvania 19104-2685
> USA
> Telephone: (215) 386-5900
> Cable: EDCOUNCIL PHA
> TELEX: 710-670-1020 (ECGMG PHA)
> Internet: http://www.ecfmg.org

REQUIREMENTS FOR INTERNATIONAL MEDICAL GRADUATE APPLICATION TO UNITED STATES RESIDENCY POSITIONS

As of July 1, 1998, new requirements went into effect for graduates of foreign medical schools to become eligible for certification by the ECFMG, as follows:

1. Passing the basic medical and clinical science components of the medical science examination within a seven year period.
2. Passing the English language proficiency test.
3. Passing the Clinical Skills Assessment (CSA), which includes an assessment of spoken English proficiency. This one-day exam evaluates your ability to gather and interpret clinical patient data and to communicate effectively in English. Over the

course of the five-hour CSA, examinees will encounter 10 standardized patients, with cases representing the broad spectrum of major clinical disciplines.

4. Documenting the completion of all requirements for, and receipt of, the final medical diploma.

Please note that students and graduates of foreign medical schools must have passed *all* examinations necessary for certification by the ECFMG by the February deadline for submission of rank lists in order to remain in the NRMP Match. The NRMP will contact the ECFMG directly to confirm that Match participants have passed the necessary examinations.

For more details on all of the above, we encourage you to read carefully the ECFMG's *Information Booklet-ECFMG Certification* which is published annually (1).

In addition to meeting the preceding general requirements for applying to residency training programs within the United States, we strongly recommend that IMGs contact the individual licensing board within each state to which they are applying for residency positions. Each state's licensing board may establish its own regulations concerning postgraduate training requirements and license eligibility, and these regulations are subject to change without notice. A complete list of the names, addresses, and phone numbers of each state's licensing board can be obtained by contacting:

> The Federation of State Medical Boards
> 400 Fuller Wiser Road
> Suite 300
> Euless, Texas 76039
> USA
> (817) 868-4000
> Internet: www.fsmb.org

For those international medical graduates who will be applying to residency programs that participate in the Electronic Residency Application Service (ERAS), your ERAS applications will be administered by the ECFMG. Additional information and ERAS application materials may be obtained through the following address:

> ECFMG *ERAS Program*
> P.O. Box 13467
> Philadelphia, PA 19101-3467
> USA
> Telephone: (215) 386-5900
> FAX: (215) 222-5641
> Internet: http://www.ecfmg.org/erasinfo.htm

With all of the preceding requirements satisfied, IMGs may have good chances of securing residency positions in specialty areas that have far more positions available than are filled each year. Alternatively, it is highly unlikely in the more competitive specialties (e.g., neurosurgery, orthopedics) that an IMG will obtain a position unless the applicant has specific personal recommendations from someone in the program, or unless his or her medical school has a relationship with a U.S. program that is promoting an international educational exchange.

ADDITIONAL TIPS FOR THE FOREIGN MEDICAL GRADUATE

If you are unable to obtain copies of the National Resident Matching Program (NRMP) application materials, you may request them through the following address:

> National Resident Matching Program
> 2501 M Street, Suite 1
> Washington, DC 20037-1307
> Telphone: (202) 828-0522

You may request information for purchasing copies of the American Medical Association's annual Directory of Graduate Medical Education Programs through the following address:

American Medical Association
Order Department-OP 416796
P.O. Box 7046
Dover, DE 19903
USA
1-800-621-8335

Foreign nationals are responsible for fulfilling the requirements for obtaining the appropriate visas in order to participate in ACGME-accredited training programs. You may request information on the Exchange Visitor Sponsorship Program (J-1 Visa) through the following address:

ECFMG Exchange Visitor Sponsorship Program
P.O. Box 41673
Philadelphia, PA 19101-1673
USA
Telephone: (215) 662-1445
FAX: (215) 386-9766

It is imperative that the IMG submit readable documents in English, utilizing the Universal Residency Application Form or other matching program application forms as requested by each individual program, or by submitting your application as indicated via the Electronic Residency Application Service (ERAS) through the ECFMG. It should go without saying that all materials submitted should be neatly typed or printed (see guidelines for the application process as outlined in Chapter 5).

Applicants may obtain current information about the status of their application to the Match in numerous ways, including the United States mail, FAX, telephone, the NRMP web site, and NRMP Voice Response System, as follows (2):

National Resident Matching Program
2501 M Street, N.W. Suite 1
Washington, D.C. 20037-1307

FAX: (202) 828-4797
Phone: (202) 828-0566
Web site: www.aamc.org/nrmp
Voice Response System (VRS): (202) 828-0566

In late 1989, the American Medical Association (AMA) reminded all directors of residency training programs of their responsibility to evaluate all applicants carefully on the basis of their individual qualifications, in consideration of their knowledge, skill, and performance. The AMA House of Delegates adopted a policy that explicitly states that it is inappropriate to measure the quality aspect solely on the basis of the country in which the medical education is received (3). With this in mind, it is extremely difficult for a residency program director to screen and interpret the credentials of all IMGs who are applying with such varied backgrounds. Most program directors will have little knowledge about the IMG's level of competency upon completion of her or his undergraduate medical education, especially when considering that the IMG's training may be from one of a myriad of educational systems around the globe. Therefore, it becomes increasingly important for the IMG to obtain constructive letters of recommendation from United States sources, which might be more easily interpreted by United States program directors.

It is also important that the applicant be available to interview, as most programs now require a personal interview.

Please note that some Specialty Boards (for example, Ophthalmology) require trainees to have completed their PGY-1 training in ACGME-accredited programs, while others may accept foreign training at the PGY-I level. Please be sure to inquire about your Specialty Board requirements before beginning your training!

After the NRMP match, depending upon the competitiveness of the specialty, there is a fair chance that an unmatched IMG with strong credentials may secure an excellent position in a program that is unfilled by contacting individual residency program directors as outlined in the NRMP Result Book (See "Scramble Process" in Chapter 8).

REFERENCES

1. *1998 Information Booklet-ECFMG Certification,* Philadelphia, Educational Commission for Foreign Medical Graduates Publishers, 1997.
2. *NRMP Handbook for Independent Applicants,* National Resident Matching Program, Washington, D.C., 1998.
3. Sammons JH. Letter to Directors of Residency Programs. American Medical Association, November 6, 1989.

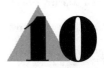

Recommended Reading

CHOOSING A SPECIALTY

1. Berg D, Cerletty J, Byrd JC. The impact of educational loan burden on housestaff career decisions. *J Gen Intern Med* 1993; 8: 143–145.
2. Calkins EV, Willoughby TL, Arnold LM. Gender and psychosocial factors associated with specialty choice. *J Am Med Wom Assoc* 1987; 42: 170–172.
3. Crandall CS, Kelen GD. The influence of perceived risk of exposure to human immunodeficiency virus on medical students' planned specialty choices. *Am J Emerg Med* 1993; 11: 143–148.
4. DeForge BR, Richardson JP, Stewart DL. Attitudes of graduating seniors at one medical school toward family practice. *Fam Med* 1993; 25: 111–113.
5. DeLisa JA, Leonard JA Jr, Smith BS, Kirshblum S. Common questions asked by medical students about psychiatry. *Am J Phys Med Rehab* 1995; 74: 145–154.
6. Dial TH, Elliot PR. Relationship of scholarships and indebtedness to medical students' career plans. *J Med Educ* 1987; 62: 316–324.
7. Dunn MR, Miller RS. The shifting sands of graduate medical education. *JAMA* 1996; 276:710–713.
8. Fincher RM, Lewis LA, Rogers LQ. Classification model that predicts

medical students' choices of primary care or non-primary care specialties. *Acad Med* 1992; 67: 324–327.

9. Fox M. Medical student indebtedness and choice of specialization. *Inquiry* 1993; 30: 84–94.

10. Gensheimer KF, Read JS, Mann JM. Physicians and medical students: factors affecting entry into public health. *Am J Prev Med* 1994; 10: 238–9.

11. Grum CM, Wooliscroft JO. Choosing a specialty: a guide for students. *JAMA* 1993; 269: 1183, 1186.

12. Henry P, Leong FT, Robinson R. Choice of medical specialty: analysis of students' needs. *Psychol Rep* 1992; 71: 215–224.

13. Herbert-Carter J. Factors influencing career choices of second-year students at a traditionally black medical school. *Acad Med* 1992; 67: 286.

14. Herold AH, Woodard LJ, Pamies RJ, Roetzheim RG, Van Durme DJ, Micceri T: Influence of longitudinal primary care training on medical students' specialty choices. *Acad Med* 1993; 68: 281–284.

15. Interspecialty Cooperation Committee. *Choosing a Medical Specialty.* Lake Forest, IL, Council of Medical Specialty Society (CMSS), 1990.

16. Iserson KV. A medical career: idealism and reality. *JAMA* 1991; 265: 1190.

17. Kassler WJ, Wartman SA, Silliman RA. Why medical students choose primary care careers. *Acad Med* 1991; 66: 41–43.

18. Kiker BF, Zeh M. Relative income expectations, expected malpractice premium costs, and other determinants of physician specialty choice. *J Health Soc Behav* 1998; 39: 152–167.

19. Lipkin M Jr, Levinson W, Barker R, Kern D, Burke W, Noble J, Wartman S, Delbanco TL. Primary care internal medicine: a challenging career choice for the 1990s. *Ann Intern Med* 1990; 112: 371–378.

20. McLaughlin MA, Daugherty SR, Rose WH, Goodman LJ. The impact of medical school debt on postgraduate career and lifestyle. *Acad Med* 1991; 66: S43–45.

21. Merrill JM, Camacho Z, Laux LF, Thornby JI, Vallbona C. Machiavellianism in medical students. *Am J Med Sci* 1993; 305: 285–288.

22. Nasmith L, Rubenstein H, Goldstein H, Sproule D, Franco ED, Tellier P. Predicting who will choose a family medicine residency. Acad Med 1997; 72: 908–912.

23. *NRMP Data—April 1998,* National Resident Matching Program, Washington, DC, 1998.

24. Potts MJ, Brazeau NK. The effect of first clinical clerkship on medical students' specialty choices. *Med Educ* 1989; 23: 413–415.

25. Richards P. *Living Medicine: Planning a Career: Choosing a Specialty.* Cambridge, Cambridge University Press, 1990.

26. Rogers LQ, Fincher RM, Lewis LA. Factors influencing medical students to choose primary care or non-primary care specialties. *Acad Med* 1990; 65(9 Suppl): S47–48.

27. Rubeck RF, Donelly MB, Jarecky RM, Murphy-Spencer AE, Harrell PL, Schwartz RW. Demographic, educational, and psychosocial factors in-

fluencing the choices of primary care and academic medical careers. *Acad Med* 1995; 70: 318–320.

28. Sakala, EP. Medical students' concerns about malpractice liability as a negative factor in specialty choice. *Acad Med* 1993; 68: 702–703.

29. Schubiner H, Schuster B, Moncrease A, Mosca C. The perspectives of current trainees in combined internal medicine–pediatrics. Results of a national survey. *Am J Dis Child* 1993; 147: 885–889.

30. Schwartz AL. Will competition change the physician workforce? Early signals from the market. *Acad Med* 1996; 71: 15–22.

31. Schwartz BS, Pransky G, Lashley D. Recruiting the occupational and environmental medicine physicians of the future: results of a survey of current residents. *J Occup Environ Med* 1995; 37: 739–742.

32. Schwartz RW, Haley JV, Williams C, Jarecky RK, Strodel WE, Young B, Griffen WO Jr. The controllable lifestyle factor and students' attitudes about specialty selection. *Acad Med* 1990; 65: 207–210.

33. Slick GL. Recruiting interns and residents to an osteopathic medical training program. *J Am Osteopath Assn* 1992; 92: 654–656.

34. Sliwa JA, Shade-Zeldow Y. Physician personality types in physical medicine and rehabilitation as measured by the Myers-Briggs Type Indicator. *Am J Phys Med Rehab* 1994; 73: 308–312.

35. Stein J. Impact on personal life key to choosing a medical specialty in the '80's. *Internal Medicine World Report* 1988; 3: 7.

36. Taylor AD. *How to Choose a Medical Specialty*. Philadelphia, W.B. Saunders Company, 1988.

37. Walters BC. Why don't more women choose surgery as a career? *Acad Med* 1993; 68: 350–351.

38. Xu G, Rattner SL, Veloski JJ, Hojat M, Fields SK, Barzanky B. The national study of the factors influencing men and women physicians' choices of primary care specialties. *Acad Med* 1995; 70: 398–404.

39. Zeldow PB, Daugherty SR. Personality profiles and specialty choices of students from two medical school classes. *Acad Med* 1991; 66: 283–287.

40. Zeldow PB, Devens M, Daugherty SR. Do person-oriented medical students choose person-oriented specialties? Do technology-oriented medical students avoid person-oriented specialties? *Acad Med* 1990; 65 (9 Suppl): S45–46.

41. Zeldow PB, Preston RC, Daugherty SR. The decision to enter a medical specialty: timing and stability. *Med Educ* 1992; 26: 327–332.

SELECTING PROGRAMS AND THE APPLICATION PROCESS

1. Aghababian R, Tandberg D, Iserson K, Martin M, Sklar D. Selection of emergency medicine residents. *Ann Emerg Med* 1993; 22: 1753–1761.

2. *A Medical Student's Guide to Strolling Through the Match*. Memphis, American Academy of Family Practice, 1990.

3. Arnold RM, Landau C, Nissen JC, Wartman S, Michelson S. The role of partners in selecting a residency. *Acad Med* 1990; 65: 211–215.

4. Baker JD III, Bailey NH, Brahen NH, Conroy JM, Dorman BH, Haynes GR. Selection of anesthesiology residents. *Acad Med* 1993; 68: 161–163.

5. Carr P, Noble J, Friedman RH, Starfield B, Black C. Choices of training programs and career paths by women in internal medicine. *Acad Med* 1993; 68: 219–223.

6. *Directory of Graduate Medical Education Programs,* American Medical Association, Chicago, annual publication.

7. Elbow P. *Writing With Power—Techniques for Mastering the Writing Process.* Oxford University Press, 1981.

8. Galazka SS, Kikano GE, Zyzanski S. Methods of recruiting and selecting residents for U.S. family practice residencies. *Acad Med* 1994; 69:304–306.

9. Grantham JR. Radiology resident selection: results of a survey. *Invest Radiol* 1993; 28: 99–101.

10. Greep NC, Rodriguez FI, Rucker L, Hubbell FA. A comparison of the methods and criteria used by traditional and primary care internal medicine programs to select residents. *J Gen Intern Med* 1995; 10:387–391.

11. Iserson KV. *Getting Into a Residency—A Guide for Medical Students.* Columbia, Camden House, Inc, 1991.

12. Kuhlmann TP, Fang WL, Fan Y. Physicians' views on how specialty-specific the first year of residency should be. *Acad Med* 1991; 66: 237–239.

13. *NRMP Directory—1999 Match,* National Resident Matching Program, Washington, DC, 1998 (annual publication).

14. *NRMP Handbook for Independent Applicants,* National Residency Matching Program, Washington, DC, 1998 (annual publication).

15. *NRMP Handbook for Students,* National Resident Matching Program, Washington, DC, 1998 (annual publication).

16. Pecora AA. Factors influencing osteopathic physicians' decisions to enroll in allopathic residency programs. *J Am Osteopath Assoc* 1990; 90: 527–533.

17. Peranson E, Randlett RR. The NRMP matching algorithm revisited: theory versus practice. National Resident Matching Program. *Acad Med* 1995; 70: 477–484; discussion 485–489.

18. Restifo KM, Tullius C. Effect of the HIV epidemic on incoming emergency medicine residents' choices of specialty and residency location. *Acad Med* 1993; 68: 931.

19. Roth AE, Peranson E. The effects of the change in the NRMP matching algorithm. National Resident Matching Program. *JAMA* 1997; 278: 729–732.

20. Simmonds AC, Robbins JM, Brinker MR, Rice JC, Kerstein MD. Factors important to students in selecting a residency program. *Acad Med* 1990; 65: 640–643.

21. Sklar DP, Tandberg D. The value of self-estimated scholastic standing in residency selection. *J Emerg Med* 1995; 13:683–5.

22. Valente J, Rappaport W, Neumayer L, Witzke D, Putnam CW. Influence of spousal opinions on residency selection. *Am J Surg* 1992; 163: 596–598.
23. Wagoner NE, Surino JR. Recommendations for changing the residency selection process based on a survey of program directors. *Acad Med* 1992; 67: 459–465.
24. Williams KJ. A re-examination of the NRMP matching algorithm. National Resident Matching Program. *Acad Med* 1995; 70: 470–476; discussion 490–494.

INTERVIEWING

1. *AMSA's Student Guide to the Appraisal and Selection of House Staff Training Programs,* 3rd edition. American Medical Student Association, 1986.
2. Batchelor AJ. The residency interview. *J Am Med Wom Assoc* 1985; 40: 42, 61.
3. Gong H Jr, Parker NH, Apgar FA, Shank C. Influence of the interview on ranking in the residency selection process. *Med Educ* 1984; 18: 366–369.
4. Regan-Smith MG, Dietrich AJ, Olson AL, Moore-West M, Argenti PA. Teaching communication and interviewing skills to medical students preparing for residency interviews. *J Med Educ* 1988; 63: 801–803.

FOR INTERNATIONAL MEDICAL GRADUATES

1. Andersen RM, Lyttle CS, Kohrman CH, Levey GS, Clements MM. National Study of Internal Medicine Manpower: XIX. Trends in internal medicine residency training programs. *Ann Intern Med* 1992; 117: 243–250.
2. Aranha GV. The international medical graduate in US academic general surgery. *Arch Surg* 1998; 133: 130–133.
3. Emson HE. Where should our new doctors come from? (letter). *Can Med Assoc J* 1993; 148: 1115; discussion 1115–1116.
4. Gary NE, Sabo MM, Shafron ML, Wald MK, Ben-David MF, Kelly WC. Graduates of foreign medical schools: progression to certification by the Educational Commission for Foreign Medical Graduates. *Acad Med* 1997; 72: 17–22.
5. Gayed NM. Residency directors' assessments of which selection criteria best predict the performances of foreign-born foreign medical graduates during internal medicine residencies. *Acad Med* 1991; 66: 699–701.
6. Greenberg DS. Cut immigration, medical schools say. *Lancet* 1996; 347: 607.
7. *1998 Information Booklet: ECFMG Certification.* Philadelphia, Educational Commission for Foreign Medical Graduates, 1997.

8. Iserson KV. *Getting Into a Residency—A Guide for Medical Students.* Columbia, Camden House, Inc., 1991.

9. Levey GS. Internal medicine and the training of international medical graduates: a time for open discussion and new approaches. *Ann Intern Med* 1992; 117: 403–407.

10. Nagral S, Lochandwala Y, Nagral A. Overseas training and doctors from developing countries (letter; comment). *Lancet* 1992; 339: 1545.

11. Part HM, Markert RJ. Predicting the first-year performances of international medical graduates in an internal medicine residency. *Acad Med* 1993; 68: 856–858.

12. Robinson BW. The oversupply of specialists and graduates of foreign medical schools (letter). *N Engl J Med* 1995; 333: 1782.

13. Romem Y, Benor DE. Training immigrant doctors: issues and responses. *Med Educ* 1993; 27: 74–82.

14. Sutnick AI, Friedman M, Wilson MP. Influence of candidates' test selections on pass rates on examinations for certification by the Educational Commission for Foreign Medical Graduates. *Acad Med* 1993; 68: 150–152.

15. Sutnick AI, Stillman PL, Norcini JJ, Friedman M, Regan MB, Williams RG, Kachur EK, Haggerty MA, Wilson MP. ECFMG assessment of clinical competence of graduates of foreign medical schools. *JAMA* 1993; 270: 1041–1045.

16. Villalona-Calero M. Pertaining for international medical graduates (letter; comment). *Ann Intern Med* 1993; 118: 397–398.

17. Weingert AL, Lynch EC. Striking "FMG" from our vocabulary (letter; comment). *Ann Intern Med* 1992; 117: 699; discussion 699–700.

18. Whitcomb ME. Correcting the oversupply of subspecialists by limiting residencies for graduates of foreign medical schools. *N Engl J Med* 1995; 333: 454–456.

19. Whitcomb ME, Miller RS. Comparison of IMG-dependent and non-IMG-dependent residencies in the National Resident Matching Program. *JAMA* 1996; 276: 700–703.